Patient-centred Ethics and Communication at the End of Life

David Jeffrey MA, FRCPE, FRCP

Radcliffe Publishing
Oxford • Seattle

Radcliffe Publishing Ltd
18 Marcham Road
Abingdon
Oxon OX14 1AA
United Kingdom

www.radcliffe-oxford.com
Electronic catalogue and worldwide online ordering facility.

British Library Cataloguing in Publication Data

A catalogue record for this book is available from the British Library.

ISBN 1 85775 621 5

Typeset by Acorn Bookwork Ltd, Salisbury, Wiltshire
Printed and bound by TJ International Ltd, Padstow, Cornwall

Contents

About the author

Dr David Jeffrey was a general practitioner in Evesham, Worcestershire for 20 years and a course organiser on the Worcester Vocational Training Scheme. In 1996 he was appointed as a consultant in palliative medicine at Cheltenham General Hospital and Honorary Senior Lecturer in palliative medicine at the University of Bristol. He retired from these posts in 2003 and is presently Chair of the Ethics Committee of the Association for Palliative Medicine for Great Britain and Ireland. He is currently working as a Consultant in Palliative Medicine in Roxburghe House, Dundee. His previous books include *There is Nothing More I Can Do* (Patten Press, 1993), *Cancer from Cure to Care* (Radcliffe Medical Press, 2000) and he is the editor of *Teaching Palliative Care* (Radcliffe Medical Press, 2002).

Acknowledgements

I would like to thank the Palliative Care Hospital Support Team at Cheltenham General Hospital, the Palliative Care Education Group for Gloucestershire (PEGG) and the Ethics Committee of the Association for Palliative Medicine for their support and encouragement. Particular thanks are due to Dr Ray Owen and Dr Colette Reid, whose wisdom informed this work.

The book would not have been possible without Pru.

Author's note

This book relates as much to nurses as it does to doctors, and has no intended gender bias. For easier reading I have referred to the healthcare professionals as 'doctors' and chosen a gender in any particular situation. Although I have drawn on the experience of others, the opinions expressed in the book are my own.

To Pru

O, but they say the tongues of dying men
Enforce attention like deep harmony:
Where words are scarce, they are seldom spent in vain;
For they breathe truth that breathe their words in pain.

King Richard II, II, i.

Introduction

The care of dying patients is a responsibility for families, healthcare professionals and society. The family and other non-professional carers provide most support in such care. Those who care face the challenge of seeing the world through the patient's eyes, as in most instances it is the patient's wishes which should direct end-of-life care. This book seeks to bridge the misunderstandings that can develop between the patient and the many individuals who care for them.

The aim of this book is to improve understanding of end-of-life issues and promote effective communication, in order to improve the care of dying patients. Although the patient with advanced cancer is the example that will be considered for our analysis, the principles and practice of care are applicable to patients with many other chronic life-threatening diseases. It is hoped that this book will interest patients and their families as well as healthcare professionals, since everyone is involved in palliative care at some time in their lives. This book aims to give professionals the confidence to involve patients in decisions that affect their care and to enable patients and their carers to understand the ethical issues involved.

Part 1 Ethics, communication and palliative care

One indicator of a civilised society is the way in which people are cared for at the end of their lives. Recent medical advances have the potential to delay death and may prolong the process of dying. This tension generates ethical dilemmas which require debate. Although the progress achieved in technological care is widely acknowledged, there are now concerns that the 'softer' psychological elements of care are neglected. In Western societies these concerns are manifested in a changing doctor–patient relationship, increasing medicalisation of death and escalating levels of patient complaints.

Medical ethics risks being perceived as a philosophical debate that is taking place on some remote level with little clinical impact. Another misperception is that ethics is limited to professional codes that determine how healthcare professionals should behave. A philosophical debate about the origins of and justifications for morality is beyond the scope of this book, but the practical application of debate and theory is an integral part of an ethical approach, as patients, families and healthcare professionals share a common purpose to care in an ethical way.

The relationship between communication, ethics and its impact on clinical care is explored. Increasing medicalisation of death and dying threatens the psychosocial elements of care, yet this care is most valuable at this stage of life. Fears, family problems and feelings of loss may surface at the end of life, causing or aggravating symptoms and suffering – a wider and subtler concept than physical pain. Relief of suffering requires psychosocial care from all carers – both family and professionals. One of the aims of palliative care is a 'good death'. In order to achieve this goal, an attempt is made to define this elusive concept.

The commonest cause of patients' complaints about their care is poor communication. Barriers to good communication are identified, and suggestions for overcoming these are discussed. Ethical dilemmas can cause distress and inhibit discussion between clinicians and patients.

Part 2 Death, dying and dilemmas

These chapters share a common format. Ethical dilemmas are illustrated by means of clinical case histories. To preserve confidentiality, these cases are an amalgam of real-life situations but do not describe any single patient's story. Following the case history, ethical issues are identified and the resulting communication problems are discussed. Practical tips are provided which may facilitate discussion and enable professionals to gain insights into the patient's world. Furthermore, patients may also gain insights into the issues that cause problems for professionals. Although all ethical and communication issues need to be addressed in an individual context, general principles may be derived, and these are summarised as key points at the end of each chapter.

Breaking bad news

The book begins by discussing the dilemmas faced by doctors and patients when cancer recurs.

Informed consent

Patients face a number of treatment options, and informed consent is a vital mechanism for protecting their autonomy from well-intentioned medical paternalism.

Stopping active treatments

The withdrawal of active treatments such as chemotherapy may be traumatic for patients and their families, who may feel abandoned. Doctors may also feel that they have failed the patient. The ethics of withholding and withdrawing medical interventions is explored in tandem with the challenge of communicating these issues in a sensitive way.

Do Not Attempt Resuscitation orders

Some patients fear the possibility of an undignified death. They may feel that, in hospital, procedures such as cardiopulmonary resuscitation will be applied whether they wish for them or not. This chapter seeks to clarify the confusion surrounding Do Not Attempt Resuscitation orders.

Feeding and fluids

Towards the end of life the withdrawal of feeding and hydration becomes controversial. Care is directed towards preserving the patient's dignity and quality of life rather than towards prolonging suffering.

Euthanasia

In reviewing the arguments with regard to euthanasia, different ways of exploring the patient's fears about their own death and dying are discussed.

Part 3 Good practice

The final part of the book is concerned with achieving good practice. At the heart of appropriate care is the patient's own experience, and their stories need to be heard if the best possible care is to be delivered. Patients differ in the extent to which they want to be involved in decision making, and different ways of exploring the extent to which patients wish to be involved in making choices are discussed.

The practice of good communication is a common theme throughout the book. Palliative care demands a multi-disciplinary team approach and this presents challenges to effective communication. Communication problems which may develop between various healthcare professionals are identified and analysed.

Education of professionals, patients and their carers is at the heart of appropriate care. The benefits of education in ethics and communication skills are identified. A study of the arts and humanities can enhance a doctor's ethical sensitivity, and ways in which a study of literature and art can improve medical decision making are suggested.

End-of-life care challenges healthcare professionals at moral and personal levels. Patients have high expectations of a 'good doctor'. The qualities required of such a doctor are discussed within a wider debate on the relevance of virtue ethics.

Part 1

Ethics, communication and palliative care

1 What is palliative care?

It seems to me most strange that men should fear;
Seeing that death, a necessary end,
Will come when it will come.

Julius Caesar, II, ii.

Case history

Mary is a 40-year-old teacher who is married to Ben, a computer programmer. They have two children, Joe (aged 15 years) and Anna (aged 12 years). Five years ago Mary developed breast cancer, which was treated by surgery, radiotherapy and chemotherapy. One year ago she had a recurrence of her cancer in her bones and lungs. She had further radiotherapy and chemotherapy. Unfortunately she had severe side-effects from the chemotherapy, including vomiting and fatigue, and was admitted to hospital with anaemia and septicaemia. She declined further chemotherapy and went home to be looked after by her general practitioner (GP) and district nurse.

Some weeks later she developed breathlessness, and her GP asked the specialist palliative care nurse (Macmillan nurse) to visit Mary and give advice regarding her further care.

The specialist nurse visited her together with Mary's own district nurse. They listened to Mary, who told them of her fears of 'choking to death'. She was also worried that she might have to return to hospital. The nurses asked whether she would like Ben to be present for the discussion of her future care. Mary agreed that she would, and together they reassured Mary that she would not be left to die in an undignified, frightening way, and that there were drugs available to alleviate her symptoms, including shortness of breath or choking feelings.

They discussed the possibility of care at home, but Ben was worried how he would cope at night if Mary's condition worsened. The district nurse told them about a Marie Curie nurse who could spend some nights with Mary in order to give Ben a rest. Mary then expressed anxiety about how her children would cope. She was told about a psychologist who was working in the local hospice who would be able to contact her and give support.

Mary deteriorated rapidly over the next two weeks, and was very sleepy. She was visited by her GP daily and had frequent visits from her district nurse and home care nurse. She died peacefully at home with Ben, Joe and Anna present.

Six months later Ben and the children saw the psychologist again for bereavement support.

Palliative care

The above case illustrates some of the characteristics of palliative care at home. The World Health Organization definition of palliative care is as follows:

> Palliative care is the active total care of patients whose disease is not responsive to curative treatment. Control of pain, of other symptoms and of psychological, social and spiritual problems is paramount. The goal of palliative care is achievement of the best quality of life for patients and their families. Many aspects of palliative care are also applicable earlier in the course of the illness, in conjunction with anticancer treatment.[1]

Palliative care developed in hospices as a response to perceived inadequacies in the care of dying patients and their families.[2] The pioneering work of hospices demonstrated that the principles of hospice care could be applied in a variety of settings – in this instance in the patient's home. Saunders and Sykes introduced the concept of 'total pain', which highlighted not only the physical aspects of the patient's pain, but also psychological, social and spiritual dimensions of the patient's distress, which can all contribute to their suffering.[3] This is well illustrated in the case history, where a symptom such as breathlessness was closely linked with both fear and fatigue. Once Mary's anxieties had been addressed, care of her symptoms became more straightforward.

Palliative care views dying as a normal process, and neither hastens nor postpones death. The multi-disciplinary team, in this case the primary care team with advice from the Macmillan nurse, provides relief from distressing symptoms by integrating the psychological and social aspects of care. In addition, it offers a support system to help patients to live as actively as possible until their death, and to help the family to cope during the patient's illness and in their own environment.

In the above definition, 'total care' refers to a holistic approach to the care of the patient. It does not mean that specialist palliative care services (in this instance the specialist nurse and psychologist) should take over the total care of the patient. Specialist palliative care services act as a resource for the patient, the family and the primary professional carers, in this case the primary care team. It may not be possible to 'control' psychological, social or spiritual problems as the definition seems to suggest, but it is important that these dimensions of care are assessed and addressed.

The scope of palliative care extends beyond the patient with a diagnosis of cancer to include patients with other chronic life-threatening diseases. Douglas challenged the hospice movement when he asked 'Why should only the minority who die of malignancies – and precious few even of them – be singled out for deluxe dying?'[4]

The view expressed above that palliative care 'neither hastens nor postpones death' reflects the philosophy of palliative care which rejects active euthanasia as a means of relieving suffering. Palliative treatments may lengthen survival, but this is not their primary goal, which is to improve quality of life.

Attempts have been made to clarify generic palliative care (or a palliative approach), and to distinguish this from specialist palliative care. A generic palliative care service consists of all the patient's and family's usual healthcare professionals who provide palliative care as an integral part of their routine clinical practice.[5]

Specialist palliative care services can be defined in terms of their core service components, their functions and the composition of the multi-professional teams that deliver the service, underpinned by the same set of principles as generic palliative care services. The components of specialist palliative care include the following:

- inpatient care
- day therapy
- bereavement services
- community care
- hospital support
- education and research.

No one individual can meet all the needs of the patient and their family. A multi-professional team delivers specialist palliative care. The specialist palliative care services include NHS and voluntary sector providers, and members of the specialist palliative care team would include the following:

- specialist nursing staff
- consultant in palliative medicine
- clinical psychologist
- social worker
- occupational therapist
- physiotherapist
- chaplain and/or other religious leaders.[5]

Palliative care in different settings

Palliative care is applicable in most settings. In the UK, almost a quarter of occupied hospital bed days are taken up by patients who are in the last year of life, and 60% of all deaths take place in hospital, despite a strong patient preference for dying at home.[6] Seymour has commented on the social isolation of dying patients in hospital, and on the failure of medical technology to coexist appropriately with dignified dying.[7] Hospital is often perceived to be a place of insecurity, discomfort, intrusion and demands for compliance.[8] This can be contrasted with the home, which is a more personal setting where there is generally a sense of social and physical security, and where sick people may have a greater sense of control. The patient's privacy can be threatened if many different professional carers visit the home in an uncoordinated manner. Patient preferences should be given attention, since it seems that so far as palliative care services are concerned the wishes of patients are at variance with the current policies.[9] By listening to patients and those close to them, the nature of appropriate care will become clear. Mola has identified the following circumstances which influence care of the dying at home:

- a favourable family environment
- acceptance of death
- a supportive family
- making the patient's preferences a priority
- availability of voluntary carers.[8]

When should palliative care start?

For cancer patients, palliative care may start at the time of diagnosis, although it is more usual to start such care when cure is no longer possible. There is a trend towards initiating palliative care earlier in the patient's illness, shifting the focus away from terminal care. This trend is linked to the desire to extend the benefits of palliative care to individuals with diseases other than cancer.[2] Currently there is confusion about the boundaries of palliative care – a specialty which relates to a stage of disease rather than to pathology – and the relationship between palliative and supportive care remains unclear. The challenge facing palliative care is how to reconcile technical expertise with demands for a humane orientation to care.[2] Psychosocial aspects of palliative care must be the concern of every member of the team, since all of the elements that contribute to 'total pain' require attention if suffering is to be relieved and quality of life improved.[10] Palliative care is not highly technological, but it is highly sophisticated and challenges practitioners on personal, clinical and ethical levels.

Key points

Palliative care:

- is concerned with quality rather than quantity of life
- addresses the needs of patients and their carers
- adopts a holistic approach
- is delivered by a multi-disciplinary team
- includes terminal care of the dying patient
- is delivered in a variety of settings.

References

1 World Health Organization (1990) *Cancer Pain Relief and Palliative Care: Report of a WHO Expert Committee*. World Health Organization, Geneva.
2 Clark D (2002) Between hope and acceptance: the medicalisation of dying. *BMJ*. **324**: 905–7.
3 Saunders C and Sykes N (eds) (1993) *The Management of Terminal Malignant Disease*. Edward Arnold, London.
4 Douglas C (1992) For all the saints. *BMJ*. **304**: 579.

5 National Council for Hospice and Specialist Palliative Care Services (2002) *Definitions of Supportive and Palliative Care. A consultation paper.* National Council for Hospice and Specialist Palliative Care Services, London.
6 Townsend J, Frank AO, Fermont D *et al.* (1990) Terminal cancer and patients' preference for place of death: a prospective study. *BMJ.* **319:** 766–71.
7 Seymour JE (2001) Critical moments – death and dying in intensive care. *J Med Ethics Med Humanities.* **3:** 8.
8 Mola GD (1997) Palliative home care. In: D Clark, J Hockley and S Ahmedzai (eds) *New Themes in Palliative Care.* Open University Press, Buckingham.
9 Clark D, Hockley J and Ahmedzai S (eds) (1997) *New Themes in Palliative Care.* Open University Press, Buckingham.
10 Sheldon F (1997) *Psychosocial Palliative Care.* Stanley Thornes Ltd, Cheltenham.

2 'I want to hold your hand'

These should be hours for necessities,
Not for delights; times to repair our nature
With comforting repose, and not for us
To waste these times.

King Henry VII, V, i.

Case history

Jim is a 20-year-old postgraduate student with advanced lymphoma that is resistant to further chemotherapy. He is dying and has only weeks to live. He is in hospital because he has asked to die in the unit where his lymphoma was treated. His parents are distressed by his pain and his sisters are at school, unable to visit as frequently as they would wish.

Jim is becoming withdrawn, and says little to the nurses or his family. A staff nurse on the haematology unit asks the palliative care team social worker to see him.

After two visits Jim confides to the social worker that he feels angry. He thinks that the doctors have let him down. He explains that he feels sad about the fact that he will be unable to complete his postgraduate diploma, and wishes that he could see more of his family without burdening them.

The social worker obtains Jim's permission to discuss these feelings of anger and isolation with his family and with a clinical psychologist in order to find ways of alleviating the situation. The psychologist is able to discuss Jim's wish to be at home without causing his family anxiety.

The social worker, family, GP and community nurses devise a package of home care for Jim and his family. This package of care is discussed with Jim, who feels much happier that he can remain at home. His pain is controlled and he spends another four weeks at home. During this time his university grants him his diploma on the basis of the work that he has completed. Jim dies at home with his family present, and the family are supported by the social worker through their bereavement.

Effective care of the dying patient needs to address the psychological and social concerns of the patient and their family. However, some authors have argued that psychosocial care is not such an integral goal of palliative care, but rather that it forms an *extrinsic* aim of care.[1] It is necessary therefore to define psychosocial care and its relationship to the palliative care of dying patients.

The National Council for Hospice and Specialist Palliative Care Services (NCHSPCS) has defined psychosocial care as:

> concerned with the psychological and emotional well-being of the patient and their family/carers, including issues of self-esteem, insight into an adaptation to the illness and its consequences, communication, social functioning and relationships.[2]

Psychosocial care addresses the psychological experiences of loss and of facing death both for the patient and in terms of their impact on those close to the patient. The patient's spiritual beliefs and cultural values are considered alongside the social factors.

Psychosocial care covers a broad spectrum of practical, psychological and spiritual aspects of daily living. Spiritual care includes emotional support offered both by professional pastoral carers and by relatives and friends in an informal way.[2] Those who deliver psychosocial care may be affected by their experiences and also require support.

Psychosocial care embraces all modes of communication that enable patients and those close to them to express feelings and concerns relating to the illness. In addition, this care offers interventions to improve the psychological well-being of the patient and their family.

In the past there has been a greater emphasis on psychological needs than on social needs.[3] The NCHSPCS guidelines emphasise the importance of social care to patients:

> The social fabric of their lives is central to how they make sense of their illness experiences, the meanings they draw upon to understand these and the range of resources they can call upon to help them manage them.[3]

It is now accepted that palliative care services do not adequately reach disadvantaged sectors of our society. Social aspects of palliative care are often limited to a focus upon the patient's family, ignoring community influences.

The NCHSPCS discussion paper suggests that the term 'psychosocial care' may be replaced by the terms 'psychological care' and 'social care' to emphasise the importance of social care, including issues of culture and ethnicity.[4]

Patients like Jim may feel a sense of loss of control, fear or anger when confronted by a terminal illness. Their relatives may also be experiencing these emotions and feel distanced from the patient. By helping patients and families to express their emotions, fear and anxiety can be reduced and family relationships improved. Spiritual issues extend beyond the religious to include existential issues relating to the meaning of an individual's life. Giving people the opportunity to express their feelings empowers them to exercise choice. Good psychosocial care within palliative care depends upon effective teamwork. Individual members of the team have overlapping roles, each profession bringing its own skills to focus on both the patient's and the family's experiences.

The boundaries of psychosocial care are unclear. For example, physical care such as washing and bathing a patient may have effects on the patient's mood, self-esteem and feelings of dependency.[2] Similarly, attending to a practical concern such as making a will may lead to a reduction in anxiety. Medical professionals in the team tend to be involved in questions of clinical care, but there is less definition of roles when confronting existential questions such as 'Why me?'. There needs to be a close collaboration between psychological and spiritual carers, as the patient may address any member of the team with such issues.

Supportive care

The development of the NHS Cancer Plan resulted in the separation and definition of the terms *palliative care* and *supportive care*, these being terms used to reflect the holistic and multi-professional dimensions of this area of care.[5] The purpose of the Cancer Plan is to ensure that people with cancer receive the appropriate professional support and care as well as the best treatment. The Cancer Plan envisaged the development of Palliative and Supportive Care Networks which corresponded to Cancer Networks.[5] The debate has now moved to differentiating between supportive and palliative care.[6]

Defining supportive care

Supportive care is designed to help the patient and their family to cope with cancer and its treatment at all stages of the cancer journey. It helps the patient to maximise the benefits of treatment and to live as well as possible with the effects of the disease.[6]

Supportive care, like palliative care, consists of a focus on quality of life, a holistic approach, and involvement in care which includes both the patient and those who matter to the patient. It values respect for patient autonomy and choice and it emphasises open and sensitive communication.[6] The similarities between the definitions of palliative and supportive care can lead to confusion.

Supportive care is principally concerned with information provision, integrated support services, patient empowerment and continuity of care, and it addresses psychological, social and spiritual needs.

Psychosocial assessment

Patients and their families face a range of issues which are not only related to illness and approaching death. The healthcare professionals need to assess individual strengths and coping styles. They also need to consider the patient's and family's previous experience of loss.

The initial assessment of a patient is conducted by a member of the specialist palliative care team, and will include a detailed medical/nursing assessment of the needs both of the patient and of the family/carers. The time invested in this initial assessment builds a firm foundation for the patient–professional partnership. The initial consultation may indicate the need for more formal psychological or social assessment.[2,7]

A psychosocial assessment examines the ways in which the illness has changed the life of the individual, and considers their coping strategies and sources of support. Discussion of hopes and expectations identifies any unfinished business. The impact of the disease on relationships and concepts of body image may identify psychosexual issues that may need to be addressed. There is also a need to identify the losses incurred in the present illness in the context of those incurred by previous bereavements. The assessment includes a discussion of the meaning of the illness both to the patient and to the family, and a review of their hopes and fears for the future.

Much of the information about the family history can be summarised on a genogram or family tree, which helps to give an insight into how the family functions and any potential conflicts, and also identifies vulnerable individuals. The team members attempt to understand the family roles and how these may have changed as a result of the illness.

Provision of practical support may allow individuals with physical needs to have the option of being discharged from hospital, or even to avoid the need for inpatient care altogether. This family perspective is placed in the context of the community, taking account of ethnic, cultural and religious factors.

Screening and assessment scales

A number of assessment scales exist that measure specific aspects of psychological symptoms or quality of life, such as the Hospital Anxiety and Depression Scale (HAD)[8] and overall Quality-of-Life Scales.[9] The patient's involvement is central, as they are the expert on what factors improve the quality of their life. There are methodological problems in assessing and measuring quality of life in patients with advanced cancer. Although the range of current measures provides researchers and clinicians with a choice, the existence of so many different assessment scales reflects an underlying methodological uncertainty.

Psychosocial interventions

Healthcare staff should all provide psychosocial care in the broad sense – psychosocial support means care that enhances well-being, confidence and social functioning. Specialist psychosocial care is provided within specialist palliative care services by staff who are appropriately trained and qualified with regard to both psychosocial assessments and interventions. Psychologists, social workers and counsellors provide psychosocial and practical care and advice, or supervision of psychosocial care by other healthcare professionals.[2]

Psychological interventions

Psychological interventions range widely from support aimed at relieving symptoms such as anxiety or anger, to the recognition and treatment of specific psychiatric disorders such as depression. These interventions may be offered to the patient, the family or bereaved individuals, to improve the psychological and emotional well-being of the patient and their family and/or carers.

The team may suggest possible interventions to the patient and family, but there is a need to be sensitive to the patient's view, which may differ from that of the professionals.

Psychological therapies are increasingly being employed in palliative care. Techniques such as cognitive behavioural therapy have been adapted from the arena of mental health for use in cancer patients who are not mentally ill but are suffering from anxiety, low mood or stress.[10] These therapies explore and seek to encourage the use of the patient's existing coping strategies. Guided imagery and patient narratives are other techniques used to aid relaxation or to gain an understanding of the patient's world.[11]

Social interventions

Specialist social workers in the team work with the patient, their family and carers within the local community. They may provide a variety of services, acting as a patient advocate to access financial or legal advice, or liaising between statutory and voluntary agencies.

Organising packages of care at home or negotiating placement and securing funding for residential/nursing home care are a familiar part of the social worker's role, but their skills extend into other areas, such as identifying people at special risk during bereavement and ensuring appropriate support.[2]

The blurring of roles is one feature of multi-professional teamworking, and this is particularly pertinent to the provision of psychosocial care. For example, bereavement support of the family may be undertaken by a social worker, a clinical psychologist or the clinical nurse specialist. It is therefore necessary to coordinate care in order to minimise the risk of the patient or their family becoming overwhelmed by support.

Staff support

The overlapping boundaries of psychosocial care may cause difficulties for professionals within the team, with the risk of some members feeling undervalued. Gaining insights into the specific needs of the individual patient requires an effort of empathy. The needs and fears of patients who are facing death make professionals feel vulnerable and inadequate. A psychological challenge for professionals is to learn to live with these negative feelings while continuing to support the patient and their family and/or carers.[10]

Managers can play a role in ensuring that there are adequate resources in terms of accommodation, administrative staffing levels, and annual and study leave to support professional teams. Increasing stress leads to absenteeism and even 'burnout'. Skilled professionals need to be valued by provision of leadership, debriefing sessions, individual supervision and appraisal, and such support structures should include volunteers.

Psychiatry and palliative care

A psychosocial assessment should distinguish between an appropriate emotional response to a life-threatening illness and the symptoms of a psychiatric disorder. Specialist psychiatric help may also be required to treat patients with existing psychiatric disorders who then develop a terminal disease.

Depression is the most commonly encountered psychiatric problem in the palliative care setting, but its definition as a diagnostic treatable clinical syndrome is not clear-cut. It may be simpler to regard the severity of depression as a continuum, with a threshold existing along this continuum of symptoms, beyond which clinicians will instigate treatment. More effective methods of diagnosing depression are needed in palliative care. Professionals need to be alert for symptoms of depression, particularly in younger patients with advanced disease.[12] Depression in patients with advanced cancer tends to be under-diagnosed and may not be appropriately treated, thus impairing the patient's quality of life. Both psychological and pharmacological treatments are effective in patients with severe depression.[10]

Why is psychosocial care so important?

The psychosocial needs of the patient and their carers require careful assessment so that appropriate levels of support and treatment can be offered. A psychosocial approach is a patient- and family-centred approach and represents a mechanism for retaining the holistic approach of modern palliative care. Psychosocial care can restore many of the original values and vision of palliative care to a specialty that is being increasingly threatened by advances in medical technology.

Clark identifies four key strands in modern palliative care:[13]

1 a shift in the literature on care of the dying from anecdote to systematic observation and research
2 a new openness about the terminal condition of patients
3 an active rather than passive approach to care of the dying
4 a growing recognition of the interdependency of mental and physical distress, notions of suffering and the concept of total pain.

It is ironic that just when it seems that palliative care has persuaded doctors to be open to an acceptance of death, the influence of advancing medical technology has led to the increasing use of futile treatments. There now appears to be an assumption in society that every cause of death can be resisted, postponed or avoided. The integration of specialist palliative care into mainstream medicine results in a biomedical model replacing the holistic caring approach. In a biomedical model suffering is equated with symptoms, the focus of care is the malfunctioning of organs, and there is a perceived need for pharmacological control of symptoms.[13]

Nowadays even the concept of 'total pain', which was intended to emphasise the holistic approach, risks being split into component parts, with integrated teamworking being replaced by specialists working in disparate roles, the consultant prescribing pain relief, the social worker dealing with patient finances, the nurse delivering physical care and the psychologist attending to the patient's worries.[14] However, the complex nature of suffering demands an integrated team approach to support and care.

Key points

Psychosocial care:

- is concerned with the psychological and emotional well-being of the patient and their family
- is an integral part of holistic palliative care
- is concerned with the appropriate use of practical resources
- depends upon a skilled assessment of needs
- delivers appropriate care in an attempt to meet identified needs
- respects a patient's autonomy and privacy
- addresses the concept of suffering and enhances simplistic biomedical models of care.

References

1 Randall F and Downie RS (1998) *Palliative Care Ethics. A good companion.* Oxford University Press, Oxford.

2 National Council for Hospice and Specialist Palliative Care Services (1997) *Feeling Better: psychosocial care in specialist palliative care.* Occasional Paper Number 13. National Council for Hospice and Specialist Palliative Care Services, London.

3 National Council for Hospice and Specialist Palliative Care Services (2000) *What Do We Mean By 'Psychosocial'?* Briefing Number 4. National Council for Hospice and Specialist Palliative Care Services, London.

4 National Council for Hospice and Specialist Palliative Care Services (1995) *Opening Doors: improving access to hospice and specialist palliative care services by members of the black and ethnic minority communities.* Occasional Paper Number 7. National Council for Hospice and Specialist Palliative Care Services, London.

5 Department of Health (2000) *The NHS Cancer Plan.* The Stationery Office, London.

6 National Council for Hospice and Specialist Palliative Care Services (2002) *Definitions of Supportive and Palliative Care. A consultation paper.* National Council for Hospice and Specialist Palliative Care Services, London.

7 Monroe B (1998) Social work in palliative care. In: D Doyle, G Hanks and N MacDonald (eds) *Oxford Textbook of Palliative Medicine.* Oxford University Press, Oxford.

8 Hoptopf M, Chidgey J, Addington-Hall J *et al.* (2002) Depression in advanced disease: a systematic review. Part 1. Prevalence and case finding. *BMJ.* **316:** 771–4.

9 Morgan G (2000) *Assessment of Quality of Life in Palliative Care.* Heinemann Medical, Oxford.

10 Chochinov HM and Breitbart W (2000) *Handbook of Psychiatry in Palliative Medicine.* Oxford University Press, Oxford.

11 Kearney M (1992) Image work in a case of intractable pain. *Palliat Med.* **2:** 152–7.

12 Lloyd-Williams M and Friedman T (2001) Depression in palliative care patients – a prospective study. *Eur J Cancer Care.* **10:** 270–74.

13 Clark D (2002) Between hope and acceptance: the medicalisation of dying. *BMJ.* **324:** 905–7.

14 Dunlop R and Hockley J (1997) A critique of the biomedical model for palliative care. In: D Clark, J Hockley and S Ahmedzai (eds) *New Themes in Palliative Care.* Open University Press, Buckingham.

3 A 'good death'

When clouds appear, wise men put on their cloaks;
When great leaves fall, the winter is at hand;
When the sun sets, who doth not look for night?
King Richard III, II, iii.

Case history[1]

Miss Smith, aged 80 years, was admitted to hospital after a stroke. She waited on a trolley in the Accident and Emergency department for six hours. On one side of her a drunk snored loudly, while on the other a confused old man tugged at his catheter.

The house officer requested a full range of investigations, including an urgent CAT scan. Despite the fact that Miss Smith was unable to speak, the house officer asked her whether she wanted to be resuscitated in the event of a cardiac arrest. The registrar asked her niece the same question, indicating that he felt her aunt should be given every chance. Her niece agreed that her aunt should be resuscitated.

Miss Smith was moved to an acute ward. Her CAT scan revealed a parietal infarct, so she was started on heparin pending oral anticoagulation when her swallowing had been assessed.

She was thirsty and fell out of bed while trying to reach a jug of water. She then became increasingly drowsy, and a second scan confirmed a subdural haematoma. The managers were anxious that the Trust might be held liable for inadequate supervision leading to the fall. It was decided to contact a neurosurgical unit for evacuation of the haematoma.

While these arrangements were being made, Miss Smith had a cardiac arrest. During cardiopulmonary resuscitation several costal cartilages gave way. She recovered enough to be aware of severe chest pain. She was transferred to the intensive therapy unit for ventilation. Later that day she was transferred to the neurosurgical unit but died in the ambulance. She was confirmed dead on arrival at the neurosurgical centre, despite further resuscitation attempts.

Defining a 'good death'

Palliative care is dedicated to improving the patient's quality of life. However, during the terminal phase of this care the aim becomes directed towards the achievement of a 'good death'. People have different views on what constitutes a good death, making it difficult to define this term. Perhaps one way to understand the meaning of a good death is to look at the factors that characterise 'bad deaths'.

Sadly, the case history above, described by McGouran, will be familiar to anyone working in an NHS hospital. It illustrates how well-intentioned but inappropriate care can lead to a 'bad death'.[1] A 'bad death' may involve 'dying alone, in pain, terrified, mentally unaware, without dignity or feeling alienated'.[2] The quality of the dying process is difficult to assess, as research in this area is sparse. However, many professionals and relatives intuitively feel that some patients die a 'bad death'.[3,4] This widespread unease has been expressed as follows: 'most doctors have witnessed patients die undignified, soulless, high-tech deaths and hoped for something better for themselves and their patients'.[5]

In contrast, Neuberger reminds us that where palliative care is available, standards of care are high: 'I do not understand why we do not celebrate the fact that we can, at best, provide a "good death" wonderfully well in this country, perhaps better than anywhere else'.[6] Good palliative care in the terminal phase strives to ensure dignity and comfort during the dying process. This approach must not be confused with euthanasia, which is concerned with the deliberate ending of a patient's life.

Dignity

Each individual has their own perception of what gives them dignity, but the concept usually conveys ideas of self-respect. Loss of body image, dependency, hospital inpatient care and unrelieved pain can all be linked to a loss of dignity. These determinants are not fixed, but may change as the person approaches death. However, dignity is common to any factors which ensure a good death.

Dignity is implicated in the manner of treating patients as well as in the manner of their dying.[7] Research on patients' perceptions of dignity is needed in order to determine the extent to which there is a significant loss of dignity in the process of dying.[8]

Suffering

Suffering is another subjective concept encompassing factors which diminish quality of life, a perception of distress, and ultimately an expression of a life not worth living.[9] Suffering is not confined to the patient, but may include the family and the healthcare professionals.

A 'good death'

The issues involved in achieving a 'good death' demand debate between patients, professionals and society. The important factors that ensure a 'good death' can be summarised as follows:

- control of pain[2]
- preparation for death[2]
- control over decisions[10]
- psychosocial, cultural and spiritual perspectives[11]
- good communication.[4,12]

Control of pain

Pain control and symptom control are realistic goals for the majority of patients. The details of appropriate prescribing are beyond the scope of this book, but the principles are simple.[13] Management plans are tailored to the individual; with a careful assessment to determine the causal factors and the impact of symptoms on the patient's life. A reassessment of symptoms is conducted if there is no response to treatment.

Palliative care depends upon anticipation of potential difficulties, with strategies being put in place to cope with problems as they occur. Patients and their families require time to come to terms with what is happening to them and to make informed choices. The drugs are simple to use, but the skill lies in attention to detail. The healthcare professional must see beyond the 'brave face' and be ready to encourage the patient to raise any concerns they may have. However, there is still a failure to relieve pain and other distressing symptoms.[14] There are many possible reasons for this, including inadequate pain assessment, insufficient use of analgesics, lack of continuity and neglect of psychosocial issues.

Preparation for death

The quality of dying can be improved if patients are aware of their situation.[15] Healthcare professionals may try to prepare the patient for the end of their life, but they may be unable to assimilate the information quickly enough to match the speed of disease progression, or they may remain in denial.[16] If the patient is unaware of the imminence of death, they may request inappropriate investigations or treatments.

In the case described above, the patient had little chance to assimilate what was happening, and progressed from one intervention to another. Acute hospital care has a momentum of its own. A study of dying patients in the USA, where terminal care is more aggressive than in the UK, concluded that 'dying patients were caught up in a medical juggernaut driven by a logic of its own, one less focused on human suffering and dignity than on the struggle to maintain vital functions'.[17]

Healthcare professionals may find it difficult to diagnose that a patient is dying. Such uncertainty should be discussed with the patient, rather than raising false hopes. The patient may lose trust in their professional carers as they continue to become weaker while receiving no acknowledgement of their deterioration.[4]

In hospitals, professionals may wish to pursue investigations, treatments or invasive procedures in a futile attempt to prolong life, since there are many situations where the future is difficult to predict. If patients are made aware of the likelihood of their dying, there is an opportunity for them to complete unfinished business, to reflect on their lives and to find some meaning for their experience.

The professional carers also need to assess the family's views of the patient's condition. The involvement of a psychologist or social worker with the relevant expertise can be invaluable in helping to meet the needs of children facing bereavement. The family may still hope and believe that their relative will recover, and gentle questioning of this view may allow them to express their real anxieties and fears. Effective communication will prepare relatives for the death and will give them a chance to say goodbye. Many bereaved relatives bitterly regret 'not being told that their loved one was dying'.[4]

Control of decisions

People like to feel in control of their lives, and such autonomy is reflected in their wish for control over the manner of their dying. In some cases this urge for control is linked to the fear of dying badly and is articulated as a request for euthanasia (*see* Chapter 11).

Patients may wish to have the opportunity to choose whether to die at home, in hospital or in a hospice. Although many express a wish to die at home, the majority of patients die in hospitals.[4] Patients should feel free to change their minds as their circumstances change, and healthcare professionals need to check whether decisions that were made at an earlier stage in the disease still apply. The fact that patients often change their minds is one of the reasons why advance directives or 'living wills' may be difficult for professionals to interpret.

Some patients fear that their lives may be prolonged pointlessly by over-enthusiastic use of medical technology.[18] Individuals may differ in their assessment of whether a treatment is futile, depending on the desired outcome and the probability of success. An individual's expectations of treatment may be influenced by their place of care. In the case described above, Miss Smith might have had a better death if she had been admitted to a community hospital and cared for by her general practitioner.[1]

The doctor's view of futility may differ from that of the patient, who may imagine a treatment to be beneficial. 'Futile' treatments require further definition. Should the view of the dying patient take precedence over the views of the healthcare professional?[19] The continued use of technical treatments needs to be considered during the care of a dying patient. Ideally the patient should have an opportunity to decide about future treatments before they become so ill that they cannot make their wishes known.

Psychosocial and spiritual perspectives

Some of the factors that characterise a good death may depend on the patient's society and culture. In a multicultural society, this mix of the norms for a good death presents a challenge to healthcare professionals. Reflecting on one's past life when approaching death is common to people from many cultures. Practitioners need to be aware of the patient's background but at the same time avoid making assumptions about their beliefs and customs. Many of the customs to which people return as they approach death have more to do with the community they come from than with their beliefs.[6]

The social concepts that characterise a good death have changed. The emphasis on an individual death is being replaced by a trend towards a shared experience with fellow sufferers.[11] In some societies, a prolonged dying process creates problems for the patient and their carers. Cultural norms range from an autonomy-centred model of a good death in Holland, to family-based care in many parts of Asia, or the hierarchical model in Japan.[11] In the autonomy-based approach favoured in many Western countries, the right of individuals to make their own choices about how they should die is often articulated as the 'right to die'. In Holland and Belgium this 'right' has grown to allow a choice about the timing of one's death (see Chapter 11). Personal preferences with regard to the mode of dying vary, some individuals preferring a quick death with no awareness of the dying process, while others prefer to have time for preparation. Medical treatments have prolonged the period for which people survive in the knowledge that they will not recover. Although this awareness has many positive aspects, it may also involve burdens, including a dread of the dying process. Patients' stories about this dilemma give insights into coping with an incurable life-threatening disease.[20]

The ethos of specialist palliative care depends on a holistic approach delivered by a multi-disciplinary team. There is a risk that psychosocial and spiritual care is neglected in the drive to specialise.[2,6] Illich has criticised the narrow 'biomedical' model of care and highlighted its deficiencies in relation to its impact on the dying process. He warned that one consequence of the medicalisation of death is that people become unable to accept death and suffering as meaningful aspects of life. Furthermore, a purely 'medical' approach risks neglecting both family care and cultural aspects of death and dying.[21]

Good communication

Good communication skills are essential in the care of the dying. The end of life offers a last opportunity to exercise choice, and such choices would be meaningless unless patients were informed by an honest discussion of their situation. Giving information at a pace that matches the patient's needs is a powerful way of showing respect for their autonomy. Healthcare professionals need to facilitate debate over the events surrounding death; such discussion is often difficult for the patient, relatives and professionals alike.[22] A high level of communication skills is needed in order to pick up subtle cues from the patient, to listen, and to use silence effectively. Such skills are not necessarily intuitive, and they can be learned.[23] It may be difficult to know whether the patient wishes to discuss death and dying. Randall and Downie warn that 'it is disrespectful of patient autonomy to embark on personal discussions unless the patient has indicated a desire or at least a willingness to do so'.[24] However, there is evidence that patients often do not raise emotional or spiritual concerns spontaneously.[25] While respecting the patient's privacy, the healthcare professional needs to encourage them to express concerns if they wish to do so.

The professionals determine how to act when the patient is no longer able to make choices because they are unconscious or too weak to communicate. The professionals' decision making may be informed by earlier discussions with the patient, when they were competent to make these important choices. The central problem in this area is a reluctance to face issues of death and dying at an earlier stage of the disease. If patients were encouraged to engage in open discussion of their wishes concerning their end-of-life care, there would be less uncertainty. Relatives would also be spared the distress of trying to guess the dying person's wishes. Healthcare professionals may seek the relatives' view as to what the patient would have wished, but no relative can give consent on another adult's behalf. Such discussions with relatives may be very difficult, and can deteriorate into a confrontation if a distressed relative demands futile treatments.

Advance directives and 'living wills' are mechanisms whereby some patients try to make their wishes known in the event of their being unable to do so at some future date. However, they are a poor substitute for honest communication at an earlier stage of the disease. The concept of dying may not be within the patient's decision-making process because they have not come to terms with the terminal nature of their condition, in which case it will be impossible for them to make rational, informed choices.[10]

There is a sense of unease with the Western medical approach to dying. Society needs to recognise that talking about death and dying is important and not something to be regarded as 'morbid'.[26] Healthcare professionals have their own fears of death, and unless they are supported they will find it difficult to help the dying and bereaved. Good communication between healthcare professionals and their patients is of paramount importance, but a high standard of communication between team members is also essential. Not surprisingly, doctors have identified communication with colleagues as one of the most stressful areas of their practice.[27]

Part of a specialist palliative care team's role is to support colleagues. All members of the team should be made aware of when a patient is likely to die, so that the patient and the relatives receive consistent messages.[4]

Quality of dying

Healthcare professionals need to reconcile the public's high expectations of technical expertise with their calls for a humane orientation with regard to care.[2] There is no single solution to achieving a 'good death', but making care of the dying a priority for healthcare would be an important first step.

Better data on how people die and patients' views on dying are needed in order to improve the care of the dying. Recent initiatives in the education of healthcare professionals include studying the medical humanities to find ways of seeing death from the patient's perspective. The Gold Standards Project is one way to improve care for the dying at home.[28] This project incorporates the use of an integrated care pathway which encourages an open attitude to death.[4] Education of healthcare professionals at all levels of their training is imperative. Medical undergraduates should be encouraged to reflect on their views and attitudes with regard to death and dying. As a result, healthcare professionals will become better prepared for the death of their patients, will understand that a 'good death' is achievable, and will be able to balance their technical expertise with humanity.

The public need information in order to dispel common myths about the dying process. Publicity is often given to anecdotes of 'bad deaths'. Much greater attention should be given by the media to patients who die a 'good death' – a more common experience in the majority of cases.

Resources for palliative care need to be made available to enable all patients to die with dignity in the setting of their choice. Appropriate standards for care of the dying should be developed and monitored. Inappropriate measures, such as hospital 'league tables' purporting to be a mark of excellence, suggest to society that death must always be resisted, postponed or avoided. In such an environment it is not surprising that palliative care is regarded as a low priority when competing for scarce resources. This simplistic view should be refined, restoring death as an integral part of life. A 'good death' then becomes a creditable aim both for healthcare organisations and for society.

Key points

- A 'good death' is a complex concept that is determined by individual beliefs.
- Standards of terminal care are variable, and some patients do suffer a 'bad death'.
- Palliative care faces the challenge of increasing medicalisation of death and dying.
- Psychosocial and spiritual issues are central to improving care of the dying.
- A 'good death' should be an important priority for healthcare.
- Much greater attention should be given by the media to patients who die a 'good death'.

References

1 McGouran RCM (2002) Dying with dignity. *Clin Med JRCPL.* **2:** 43–4.
2 Clark D (2002) Between hope and acceptance: the medicalisation of dying. *BMJ.* **324:** 905–7.
3 Clark J (2003) Patient-centred death. *BMJ.* **327:** 174–5.
4 Ellershaw J and Wand C (2003) Care of the dying patient: the last hours of life. *BMJ.* **326:** 30–34.
5 Smith R (2003) Death, come closer. *BMJ.* **327:** 172.
6 Neuberger J (2003) A healthy view of dying. *BMJ.* **327:** 207–8.
7 Raeve L de (1996) Dignity and integrity at the end of life. *Int J Palliat Care Nurs.* **2:** 71–6.
8 Agrawal M and Emanuel E (2002) Death and dignity: dogma disputed. *Lancet.* **360:** 1197–8.
9 Cherny NI, Coyle C and Foley KM (1994) Suffering in the advanced cancer patient: a definition and taxonomy. *J Palliat Care.* **10:** 57–70.
10 Smith R (2000) A good death: an important aim for health services and us all. *BMJ.* **322:** 810–11.
11 Walter T (2003) Historical and cultural variants on the good death. *BMJ.* **327:** 218–20.
12 Sternhauser KE, Clipp EC, McNeilly M *et al.* (2000) In search of a good death: observations of patients, families and providers. *Ann Intern Med.* **132:** 825–32.
13 Doyle D and Jeffrey D (2000) *Palliative Care in the Home.* Oxford University Press, Oxford.

14 Edmonds P (2003) If only someone had told me . . . A review of the care of patients dying in hospital. *Clin Med*. **3**: 149–52.

15 Seale C *et al.* (1997) Awareness of dying. *Soc Sci Med*. **45**: 477–80.

16 Finlay I (1996) Difficult decisions in palliative care. *Br J Hosp Med*. **56**: 264–7.

17 Moskowitz EH and Nelson JL (1995) The best laid plans. *Hastings Center Rep*. **Nov–Dec**: 53–5.

18 Age Concern (1999) *Debate of the Age Health and Care Study Group. The future of health and care of older people: the best is yet to come.* Age Concern, London.

19 Finlay I (2003) Dying with dignity. *Clin Med JRCPL*. **3**: 102–3.

20 Picardie R (1998) *Before I Say Goodbye*. Penguin, Harmondsworth.

21 Illich I (1976) *Limits to Medicine. Medical nemesis: the expropriation of health*. Masson Boyer, London.

22 Shah S and Lloyd-Williams M (2003) End-of life decision making – have we got it right? *Eur J Cancer Care*. **12**: 212–14.

23 Fallowfield L (2003) Communication with the patient and family in palliative medicine. In: D Doyle *et al.* (eds) *Oxford Textbook of Palliative Medicine* (3e). Oxford University Press, Oxford.

24 Randall F and Downie RS (1998) *Palliative Care Ethics. A good companion*. Oxford University Press, Oxford.

25 Maguire P and Pitceathly C (2002) Key communication skills and how to acquire them. *BMJ*. **325**: 697–700.

26 Shipman C, Levenson R and Gillan S (2002) *Psychosocial Support for Dying People*. King's Fund, London.

27 Jeffrey D (2000) *Cancer: from cure to care*. Hochland & Hochland, Manchester.

28 Thomas K (2003) *Caring for the Dying at Home: companions on the journey*. Radcliffe Medical Press, Oxford.

4 Why ethics?

We are all men,
In our own natures frail, and capable
Of our flesh; few are angels.
King Henry VIII, V, ii.

Case history

Clare, a 50-year-old woman with advanced pancreatic cancer, is dying. She has been admitted to hospital for pain control, and is now bed bound and becoming weaker each day. She is intermittently confused, barely able to communicate and unable to swallow. Her pain is well controlled with analgesics administered via a syringe driver. Her son, a journalist, speaks to the doctor during an evening visit and says 'I want my mother to have drip feeding and fluids'.

How should the doctor to respond to this request?

Ethics can be perceived as an abstract philosophical discipline, shrouded in jargon and apparently out of touch with the realities of healthcare provision. However, in this book it is argued that ethics, communication and clinical medicine are inseparable, and that ethics has a central role in clinical decision making. Traditionally, healthcare demands that clinicians are competent, possess good communication skills and have an understanding of the legal dimension of any clinical situation. In addition, compassion and ethical sensitivity are needed.[1] Ethical dilemmas occur more frequently as healthcare involves increasingly sophisticated medical technology. Patients' expectations have been raised, with some imagining that doctors can postpone death almost indefinitely, while others who are wary of modern technology fear a prolonged, undignified process of dying.

In the UK, successive reorganisations of the NHS have generated a consumerist approach to healthcare, whereby the patient is viewed as a customer and patients' views of doctors have also undergone change. There is a new emphasis on the rights of patients and the duties of doctors, with less attention being paid to the responsibilities of patients and the rights of healthcare professionals.

Ethical frameworks

Ethics is a dynamic activity that involves reflecting on the wisdom of past philosophers and evaluating its relevance today. To facilitate discussion of ethical dilemmas, a straightforward ethical language is required. Ethical issues that arise during the care of patients need to be identified and frameworks developed to assist healthcare professionals and patients in decision making.[2]

Ethical practice

Utilitarianism

A brief review of ethical frameworks will begin by looking at how to achieve the best outcome or 'utility' for the majority of people. This ethical theory, which is based on the consequences of our actions, was developed by John Stuart Mill and Jeremy Bentham and is known as *utilitarianism*.[3] The consequences of our actions become of principal concern, in seeking to achieve the greatest good for the greatest number of people. There is a danger that in the attempt to maximise utility for as many as possible, an important minority might be overlooked. For example, resources for care of the dying might be diverted to patients who require active acute care. Utilitarian ethics appeals to politicians and managers who promulgate a free-market approach to healthcare.

Deontology

Healthcare professionals may find it difficult to work within a utilitarian framework, as their ethos is 'to do the best' for the individual patient. Such a duty-based approach to ethics was advocated by Kant and is known as *deontology*.[4] Kant believed that it was imperative to treat people as individuals of equal moral worth and never as a means to an end. Doctors have specific obligations and duties towards their patients, just as a father might have a duty to a son. Each individual action is subject to moral scrutiny, and intentions of a moral action are of greater significance than outcomes. In the clinical case described above, the doctor guided by deontological theory would be concerned about acting in Clare's 'best interests', and resource limitations or implications for other patients would be of less relevance.

It is easy to see how these two ethical theories may clash and cause doctors to feel uncomfortable as they try to do their best for the individual patient while at the same time feeling restricted by the wider needs of the community. These dilemmas are heightened when doctors invite patients to enter research trials which may be of little or no benefit to them but may benefit future patients.

Principles

Another approach to thinking about ethical dilemmas is based on four principles originally developed by Beauchamp and Childress to guide medical care,[5] and now widely adopted in Western countries:

- respect for autonomy (self-determination)
- beneficence (doing good)
- non-maleficence (not causing harm)
- justice (being fair).

Although these four principles provide a common set of moral issues, they do not necessarily provide ethical solutions to clinical dilemmas.[6]

Autonomy

Autonomy has been defined as 'the capacity to think, decide and act on the basis of such thought and decision, freely and independently'.[7] In expressing autonomy, an individual shapes and gives meaning to their life. A patient's autonomy may be respected in a number of ways – by telling the truth, by preserving confidentiality and by obtaining informed consent to any proposed medical intervention.[6] Respect for a patient's autonomy can only occur if healthcare professionals have good communication skills. In the above case history, in which Clare's death is (or is thought to be) imminent, respect for the patient's autonomy assumes a particular importance. In Clare's case, respecting autonomy is difficult because she is unable to communicate her decisions. Patients with cancer can appear physically frail and may fall prey to well-intentioned but unwanted medical intervention. Ethical dilemmas may be generated by this conflict between patient autonomy and medical power.

Paternalism

Paternalism is a denial of autonomy, and a substitution of an individual's judgements or action for his or her own good. A conflict may exist between a doctor's duty of beneficence (to do what is best for the patient), and their duty of respect for the patient's autonomy. A doctor has limited qualifications for weighing the various 'harms' and 'benefits' in the proposed act, whereas the patient is an expert on his or her own life. Doctors may be medical 'experts', but they are not 'experts' on the social, spiritual or emotional aspects of the patient's life. Yet these non-medical aspects may be of more significance to the patient than the illness. An essential part of the principle of autonomy is respect for the individual, who may have different priorities to those of the healthcare professional.

Paternalism seeks to treat patients – inappropriately – as children, encouraging them to become over-dependent. However, paternalism may spring from the best of motives – to act in the best interests of the patient. Patient autonomy can best be respected by providing honest information and ensuring that consent is given before any medical intervention. Informed consent acts as a mechanism to protect autonomy against paternalistic intervention in the case of patients who are able to make decisions. If patients are confused, unconscious or unable to communicate their choices, the ethical situation becomes complex and doctors may have to exercise a degree of paternalism.

Informed consent

All medical interventions – whether diagnostic, therapeutic or for research – have the potential to violate patient autonomy. The central function of informed consent is to ensure a sharing of power and knowledge between doctor and patient. A mutual understanding results from this sharing process, as patients receive appropriate care from a doctor whom they trust and respect. Doctors should offer alternatives and discuss choices, rather than making them. This 'sharing' option is clinically and emotionally more demanding for doctors, as it involves an ethical sensitivity to the changing needs of the patient. A patient may legitimately ask a doctor for her opinion as an expert: 'What would you do if you were in my situation?' If this is a request for guidance, then to give advice does not infringe on the patient's autonomy. The alternative may be to leave the patient with more uncertainty than they can endure.

Autonomy and justice

Western medical ethics favours an autonomy-based approach to healthcare that corresponds to deontological principles. An ethical framework that focuses simply on an individual's rights risks being unfair to others, as issues of autonomy may clash with principles of justice. Respect for an individual's autonomy is not an absolute principle, but is tempered by a consideration of the autonomy of others. A patient might choose autonomously to receive an expensive new chemotherapy drug, but considerations of the cost to other patients might result in the denial of treatment with this drug. There is nothing in the principle of respect for autonomy which requires that doctors must comply with every request that the patient makes.[8]

Beneficence vs. non-maleficence

'Do no harm' is a Hippocratic maxim that is instilled into every medical student. However, in order to act for the good of a patient (the duty of beneficence) doctors often cause great harm. For example, in their urge to cure a patient with breast cancer doctors may employ mutilating surgery (mastectomy), or even cause death (by neutropenic sepsis). The principles of beneficence and non-maleficence are often opposed, and a balance should be sought between the prospects of a good outcome and the risk of harm, in order to produce a net benefit for the patient. Healthcare professionals need to be able to communicate the risks and probabilities of benefit in such a way that the patient understands them and is able to make an informed choice. In this way professionals both respect and enhance the patient's autonomy with regard to making their own decision.

Ethical conflict

Although the 'four principles' assist in clarifying thinking and identifying issues, the principles may clash. The potential for conflict between the four principles may be expressed diagrammatically as shown in Figure 4.1.

In any ethical dilemma it may be difficult to decide which principle should have priority. Autonomy requires a capacity to deliberate and to reflect on choices. It is necessary to define who qualifies as an autonomous individual. How much capacity does someone need in order to be regarded as adequately

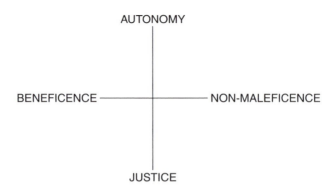

Figure 4.1 Ethical conflict

autonomous? Perhaps autonomy is only respected when patients are choosing for the 'right reasons', and is ignored when patients disagree with their doctors. In Clare's case the doctor wishes to act in her best interest, which may conflict with the son's interest. The administration of fluids and feeding may cause more harm than good, and these possibilities need to be carefully considered and balanced. In the above case history the doctor finishes her shift in ten minutes' time, and she is uncertain whether she should embark on a lengthy discussion with Clare's son or call in a colleague who does not know the patient. It is difficult to know what Clare would have wished if she had been able to choose. There is a conflict of interest between the son, who feels that he knows what his mother would have wished, and the doctor, who can see no benefit in administering the fluids. Although the doctor recognises that Clare is dying, she cannot be sure how long she might survive.

Decisions can be difficult, and an 'ethical pause' is required to enable the doctor to consider the issues with the patient, the family and other healthcare professionals. Time is required for doctors to understand the situation from the patient's perspective, and for patients to understand the choices that are available to them. By allowing this 'ethical pause', both parties come to a better understanding of each other's view and informed consent is realised.

Tavistock principles

In the search for an 'ethical compass' to guide decision making in healthcare, a multi-disciplinary group consisting of healthcare professionals, ethicists and a philosopher developed an alternative set of principles, known as the Tavistock principles.[9] These can be summarised as follows:

- **rights** – people have a right to healthcare
- **balance** – care of individual patients is central, but the health of populations is also of concern to us
- **comprehensiveness** – in addition to treating illness, we have an obligation to ease suffering, minimise disability, prevent disease and promote health
- **cooperation** – healthcare succeeds only if we cooperate with those we serve, with each other and with those in other sectors
- **improvement** – improving healthcare is a serious and continuing responsibility
- **safety** – do no harm
- **openness** – being open, honest and trustworthy is vital in healthcare.[10]

These principles, which are derived from the discussions of the Tavistock group, provide a different way of looking at ethical issues – emphasising patient involvement, multi-disciplinary teamwork and equity. Globally a right to free healthcare sadly does not exist, both in the most affluent countries and in the so-called 'Third World'. The Tavistock principles are consistent with a consumerist view of healthcare, with their emphasis on balance, comprehensiveness and improvement. By applying these principles to clinical problems, healthcare professionals can assess whether they assist decision making. However, it is unlikely that any set of principles will cover all situations. Other ethical frameworks need to be considered.

Acts and omissions

Doctors owe patients a duty not to kill them, but feel less strongly that they have to 'strive officiously to keep [them] alive'.[11] The traditional medical view that it is worse to kill than to let die reflects the Acts and Omissions Doctrine derived from Roman Catholic theology. The doctrine argues that actions which result in some undesirable consequence are morally worse than a 'failure to act' which has the same consequence. In the case described above, the doctor may withhold intravenous feeding and fluids from Clare if she feels that they would not result in a medical benefit, even if this were to shorten Clare's life. According to the arguments of Acts and Omissions Doctrine, this omission to treat is morally different and preferable to carrying out an act that would shorten Clare's life. One unfortunate consequence of this doctrine has been to confuse clinical decisions to withhold a futile treatment with decisions about euthanasia. Withholding intravenous fluids from a dying patient at the very end of life should not be regarded as euthanasia.

Double effect

In a moral analysis, a person's intentions and obligations are relevant, as are the outcomes of their actions. There is an argument that a clear distinction can be made between intended and unintended consequences of an action, known as the principle of double effect.[7] In Clare's case, a doctor who gives an injection of diamorphine with the intention of relieving the patient's pain is not morally culpable if, as a side-effect of this necessary treatment, the patient becomes weaker and develops a fatal pneumonia. This would be quite different from intentionally giving the patient a large dose of diamorphine with the intention of ending their life. The doctrine of double effect distinguishes between intended and foreseen consequences of a medical intervention.

Ordinary and extraordinary means

The primary goal of terminal care is the comfort of the patient. In deciding whether to withhold intravenous fluids and feeding of patients with advanced cancer, the doctor must consider the views of the patient and their family and assess the benefits and burdens of treatment. A theological doctrine raised in the ethical debate is that of ordinary and extraordinary means. This doctrine states that the good of saving life is morally obligatory if its pursuit is not excessively burdensome or disproportionate to the expected benefit.[7] Ordinary means (basic care such as food and water) are morally obligatory, whereas extraordinary means (such as intravenous drips) are morally optional. However, there are no clear boundaries between ordinary and extraordinary means – the burdensome quality of treatment has to be determined in each individual case, rendering this doctrine of little help in deciding whether or not a treatment should be given.

Virtue ethics

Virtue ethics is an ethical framework that emphasises the virtues or moral character, rather than rules or consequences.[12] Classic virtue theory was originally described by Plato and Aristotle, but has been revived during the last ten years. Virtue ethics addresses issues of motive, moral integrity, wisdom and emotions. It is concerned more with the moral integrity of the person than with formal moral principles, addressing the question 'What sort of person should I be?' rather than 'What sort of action should I take?'.

Aristotle's concept of practical wisdom (*phronesis*) is a core concept of virtue ethics. The character traits or virtues merge with emotions such as compassion – an essential part of the professional–patient relationship. If professionals lack compassion, they do not empathise with patients. In the case described above the doctor would be asking herself whether she was behaving in a way that concurred with the professional codes and standards of good practice of a good doctor.

Codes of conduct

Since the earliest days of medicine, codes of conduct have provided a baseline position for guiding doctors' behaviour. The ancient Hippocratic oath has been replaced by a number of different ethical codes which attempt to cover the increasingly complex judgements that a doctor must make. A code of conduct for doctors practising in the UK has been produced by the General Medical Council:[13]

The duties of a doctor[13]

Patients must be able to trust doctors with their lives and well-being. To justify that trust, we as a profession have a duty to maintain a good standard of practice and care and to show respect for human life. In particular, as a doctor you must:

- make the care of your patient your first concern
- treat every patient politely and considerately
- respect patients' dignity and privacy
- listen to patients and respect their views
- give patients information in a form that they can understand
- respect the rights of patients to be fully involved in decisions about their care
- keep your professional knowledge and skills up to date
- recognise the limits of your professional competence
- be honest and trustworthy
- respect and protect confidential information
- make sure that your personal beliefs do not prejudice your patients' care

- act quickly to protect patients from risk if you have good reason to believe that you or a colleague may not be fit to practise
- avoid abusing your position as a doctor
- work with colleagues in the ways that best serve patients' interests.

In all of these matters you must never discriminate unfairly against your patients or colleagues, and you must always be prepared to justify your actions to them.

Ethical codes are necessary and provide standards, but they lack the flexibility to be really helpful in a difficult ethical dilemma when a decision must be made.

Ethical progress

The various ethical models focus on different moral concepts – principles, virtues, consequences and duties. Each has its limitations in any ethical analysis – it may not be enough to be a 'good doctor' with practical wisdom. An ethics of 'responsibility' is a recent development that incorporates features of different ethical models.[14] Gracia's model proposes that although duty-based and virtue-based ethical models appear to be consistent with the values of palliative care, the relevance of consequences cannot be dismissed. He suggests that there is a need to combine and balance duties, principles, virtues and consequences. People who are affected by a decision about their future should be given an opportunity to participate in such a decision. Patients are respected as agents of equal moral value, with dignity. Responsibility ethics both respects and enhances autonomy without leaving the patient feeling abandoned. It fosters values that give rise to compassion and care. The 'wise' doctor can utilise different ethical frameworks to involve patients and colleagues in reaching the best possible decision. A team approach allows healthcare professionals to share problems and to coordinate skills for the benefit of the patient. There may be problems in reaching a moral consensus between team members, but it is important for the debate to take place. Someone needs to accept responsibility for the group decision.[15] The process of attempting to resolve ethical dilemmas may be stressful, particularly if the patient is unable to make choices. Those working in palliative care need mutual support and time to reflect on their practice.

Conclusions

Ethics extends beyond the narrow confines of medical bioethics. A broader perspective includes virtue ethics, which provides new insights into handling the uncertainties of end-of-life care. This expansion of ethical perspectives mirrors an ethos of palliative care that aims to adopt a holistic model of care. This form of care requires considerations beyond principilism. Dignity, quality of life, relief of suffering, and care for the carers are all embedded in palliative care ethics. Specialist palliative care is a discipline that will either become integrated into mainstream medicine or develop into a separate specialty.[8] If integration is to be the chosen route, how are the boundaries of palliative care to be defined? Palliative care has an ethos of family-centred care which challenges current ethical concepts of the primacy of patient autonomy.

Key points

A number of different ethical frameworks have been discussed:

- *utilitarianism* – any action should have the best possible consequences; the greatest good for the greatest number
- *deontology* – a duty-based theory; do unto others as you would be done by
- *principles* – autonomy, beneficence, non-maleficence and justice
- *Tavistock principles* – a more recent attempt to develop a moral compass
- *theological principles* – these are often invoked in arguments about euthanasia and withholding of futile treatments, two situations that should not be confused and which require separate debate
- *virtues* – behave in a way that characterises a good person
- *codes* – standards of practice form a baseline but do not often help to provide an answer to an ethical dilemma
- *ethical progress* – recent trends have been to amalgamate the various frameworks to guide ethical actions; responsibility ethics
- *palliative care ethics* – challenges current ethical concepts of the primacy of patient autonomy.

References

1 Hope T and Fulford KWM (1996) *The Oxford Practice Skills Course*. Oxford University Press, Oxford.
2 Jeffrey D (1993) *There is Nothing More I Can Do*. Patten Press, Penzance.
3 Mills JS (1974) Utilitarianism. In: M Warnock (ed.) *Utilitarianism*. Fontana, Glasgow.
4 Kant I (1964) Groundwork of the metaphysics of morals. In: HJ Paton (ed.) *The Moral Law*. Hutchison University Library, London.
5 Beauchamp TL and Childress JP (1989) *Principles of Biomedical Ethics* (3e). Oxford University Press, Oxford.
6 Gillon R (1994) Medical ethics: four principles plus attention to scope. *BMJ*. **309:** 184.
7 Gillon R (1985) *Philosophical Medical Ethics*. John Wiley & Sons, Chichester.
8 Clark D and ten Have H (2003) *Facing Death. The ethics of palliative care: European perspective*. Open University Press, Buckingham.
9 Smith R, Hiatt H and Berwick D (1999) Shared ethical principles for everybody in health care: a working draft from the Tavistock Group. *BMJ*. **318:** 248–51.
10 Berwick D *et al.* (2001) Refining and implementing the Tavistock principles for everybody in health care. *BMJ*. **323:** 616–20.
11 Clough AH (1977) The latest decalogue. In: J Glover (ed.) *Causing Deaths and Saving Lives*. Penguin, Harmondsworth.
12 Hursthouse R (1999) *On Virtue Ethics*. Oxford University Press, Oxford.
13 General Medical Council (2001) *Good Medical Practice*. General Medical Council, London.
14 Gracia D (2003) Responsibility ethics. In: H ten Have and D Clark (eds) *Facing Death. The ethics of palliative care: European perspective*. Open University Press, Buckingham.
15 Randall F and Downie RS (1998) *Palliative Care Ethics. A good companion*. Oxford University Press, Oxford.

5 'Why won't you listen to me?'

Give sorrow words: the grief that does not speak
Whispers the o'er-fraught heart and bids it break.
Macbeth, IV, iii.

Why do we need good communication?

Patients need to have information about the diagnosis, prognosis and treatment choices in order to be able to make autonomous choices and plan realistically for the future. They also need to be aware of the services and resources for support that are available to them and their family. This chapter identifies general principles for good communication (detailed analysis of specific issues is covered in later chapters).

Good communication skills employed by professionals can make them aware of the patient's unspoken concerns. A holistic assessment of the patient's requirements is fundamental to palliative care. Not only does skilled communication allow an exchange of information between patient and professional, but also the telling of the story is of itself of therapeutic benefit.[1,2]

Informed consent depends on honest communication between the doctor and the patient. Discussion of ethical dilemmas involves professionals, relatives and the patient, and is an essential part of a trusting relationship. Talking to relatives and to children can be particularly difficult for healthcare professionals. Multidisciplinary teamwork depends on effective communication between the professionals (*see* Chapter 13).

By communicating well, doctors can help to reduce uncertainty and try to prevent unrealistic expectations while at the same time maintaining hope. Good communication can improve the quality of dying.

In helping patients to adjust to their situation, a successful communicator needs to give time and continuity of care. Breaking bad news is difficult for both professionals and relatives, and collusion and conspiracies of silence can develop when attempts are made to shield the patient from bad news. Sometimes just sitting quietly with a distressed patient is the most supportive form of communication.

The patient may also have psychological difficulties in coping with bad news and its impact on the family. The time of diagnosis, treatment and recurrence may be associated with considerable social and psychological morbidity, which may remain unrecognised by healthcare professionals. Patients are often reluctant to disclose psychological problems, while professionals may avoid asking about them.[2]

Patients and their carers consistently identify the need for good communication with professionals, and poor communication is the commonest reason why they complain about doctors.[3]

There is a value in listening to the patient's story and helping them to place the illness in the context of their life's plan. Good communication is a fundamental part of ethics and clinical care.

Barriers to good communication

There are a number of barriers that present challenges to good communication. These will now be discussed in turn.

Lack of time

Case history

Dr Green is in the middle of a busy morning surgery. She is running 40 minutes late and has ten patients to see. Mrs Brown has been treated with radiotherapy for bone metastases from a breast cancer. Her pain is now well controlled, and she has 'popped in' for review and a further supply of analgesics. After spending ten minutes assessing her pain control and prescribing the appropriate analgesics, Dr Green suggests a follow-up appointment in two weeks' time.

Mrs Brown says 'Thank you, doctor. I was so relieved to hear from the radiotherapist that my disease is now progressing. Perhaps I won't need any more tablets in a couple of weeks'.

The general practitioner now has several problems.

- Should she explore Mrs Brown's misunderstandings?
- How will the remaining patients cope with a longer wait?
- When will she find time to do her home visits?
- How can she conceal her own feelings of stress?

A common justification for inadequate communication is lack of time. Clinicians often work with unrealistic caseloads. However, patients value the time spent with them, and their satisfaction with general practitioners and their degree of involvement in decision making are directly related to a longer consultation.[4]

Planning of workloads needs to be realistic to allow more time for patients. Resources may be better used by involving other team members. In the case described above, Mrs Brown has a good relationship with a Macmillan nurse, so one approach open to Dr Green would be to refer her to the specialist nurse for support in clarifying her misunderstandings. Early action to resolve these misunderstandings would save Dr Green time in the future.[5]

Lack of privacy

Case history

Freda, a 48-year-old woman, is in a six-bedded ward recovering from a laparotomy she underwent yesterday evening. The surgeon found widespread intra-abdominal cancer which could not be removed. He visits Freda on a ward round with a nurse, a registrar and a medical student. Freda is awake and her husband is sitting beside the bed. The curtains are drawn around the bed.

Surgeon: 'Good morning, Mrs White. How are you feeling?'
Freda: 'A bit sore ... was the operation a success?'

The surgeon now has a number of problems.

- How can he maintain confidentiality?
- What is Freda's understanding of her situation?
- Does Freda want her husband to know about it?
- How will he deal with her distress?
- What will the effect of breaking bad news be on her husband and the other patients in the ward?

Maintaining confidentiality is one way of respecting a person's autonomy, and it forms an essential part of a trusting relationship. In practice, absolute confidentiality is hard to achieve and breaches are commonplace in hospital and community settings.

Preparation is of paramount importance for good communication. To preserve confidentiality, staff need to arrange for a private space to be available for critical conversations. Provision of privacy needs a higher priority in the allocation of space in clinical areas. Patients and relatives are often expected to conduct personal conversations with healthcare professionals in open wards – a situation which would not be tolerated, for example, in a solicitor's office.

The presence or absence of relatives can create problems with regard to confidentiality. Doctors must obtain the patient's consent before disclosing confidential information to members of the family. It should not be assumed that the patient wants their relatives to be informed. The patient may be keen to have a discussion with the doctor on their own, while the relatives may feel angry if they are not included in the discussion or if the patient is given bad news when they are not present. The patient should be consulted first about whether they wish their relatives to be present. Offering them such a choice gives the patient a sign (a 'warning shot') that a serious discussion is about to take place, allowing them some time to prepare for the bad news.

Uncertainty

Case history

Dr Payne, an oncologist, says to Mrs Ash, a patient with bowel cancer, 'I'm afraid that the scan shows that the cancer has spread to your liver.' Mrs Ash asks 'How long have I got?'

The oncologist is faced with a number of potential problems.

- He does not know for certain how long she might live.
- He might distress her.
- What does the patient really want to know?

Communication is difficult for patients, relatives and professionals in uncertain situations. Patients need to have a sense of control over their life plans, but a diagnosis of cancer threatens illusions of control, and suddenly the world becomes frightening and unpredictable. Restoring a sense of control may enable patients to feel 'safe' even in a life-threatening situation. In the case described above it will be necessary to assess the patient's views of her illness and how much she wants to know about her prognosis. The information needs to be tailored to the needs of the individual. Uncertainty can be acknowledged by doctors, with discussion of fears of death or the setting of goals for a limited future being determined by the patient.

Embarrassment

Case history

Jim, a young man with lung cancer, is becoming weaker every day and is confined to bed. He talks to the district nurse while she is adjusting his syringe driver, and says 'Nurse, I am not ready to die.'

The nurse is faced with the following problems:

- talking about death and dying
- distressing the patient
- her own fears about dying
- uncertainty about the patient's prognosis
- no clear idea of the patient's fears
- not knowing what the patient has been told.

A general reluctance in society to discuss death, combined with a desire not to cause distress, can make communication between healthcare professionals and patients difficult.

Listening is the key skill in this area, where the professional needs to convey to the patient that she is approachable and empathises with his suffering. Patients do not expect healthcare professionals to have glib answers to existential questions, but they do need to have contact with another human being who is prepared to be with them and to listen to their fears.

Collusion

Case history

Anne is married to Henry, who is dying from lung cancer which has spread to his liver. A community nurse visits him at home. At the front door Anne says to her 'You are a new nurse here. It is imperative that you don't tell my husband how ill he really is ... it would kill him.'

The nurse now faces the prospect of becoming involved in a conspiracy to protect Henry from bad news. There are a number of aspects to her dilemma.

- The nurse has a duty to be honest with her patient.
- Why does Anne want to shield her husband from the truth?
- What does Henry understand about his illness?
- How has Anne come to know the situation before her husband does?
- What are the effects of this collusion on the relationship?

Collusion often occurs because relatives feel that the patient would be unable to hear the bad news without being overwhelmed by it. Protective behaviour such as this is a form of paternalism and springs from good motives. However, it is a serious breach of patient confidentiality to discuss details of a patient's case with his relatives before he has been given the information himself, so collusion with relatives is preventable.

If collusion exists, time is needed for the healthcare professional to explore the relatives' motives for maintaining the deception. It may be the first time that a healthcare professional has sat down with the relative to listen to their concerns rather than focusing on those of the patient. Relatives also need to know that the patient may be aware of the gravity of the situation but is trying to protect the family from the truth. In the case described above, the nurse can facilitate communication between Anne and Henry. Sometimes it is a doctor who initiates the collusion – there are still doctors who are perceived by colleagues as 'tellers' or 'non-tellers' of bad news.

Maintaining hope

Case history

Alfred, a 42-year-old man with bowel cancer, has been admitted from the clinic for pain control. He is quiet and withdrawn, but when a nursing auxiliary makes him a cup of tea he confides 'They have told me that they can't cure it ... there's no hope now.'

This situation is difficult for a number of reasons.

- There is a difference between hope of cure and hope for other things which make life worth living.
- Hopelessness is a risk factor for the development of depression.
- The patient may reject potentially helpful palliative interventions.
- The situation will almost certainly cause great distress to the patient's family.

One way of coping with this situation is to acknowledge the patient's distress, allow time for the shock to subside, and encourage the patient to set goals other than cure – for example, getting home to spend time with their family. The healthcare professional needs to be alert for signs of the development of clinical depression.[5]

Anger

Case history

Diana, a 40-year-old woman with advanced breast cancer, has received three different forms of palliative chemotherapy in addition to hormone therapy, surgery and radiotherapy. Her oncologist has advised her that further active treatments are no longer worthwhile because her disease is progressing despite their efforts. He suggests that she should now have specialist palliative care to keep her comfortable.

Diana shouts at him 'How dare you give up on me? What do you mean ... I'm not worthwhile? If you had been bothered to scan me earlier after my first treatment I would never have been in this situation.'

Anger directed at oneself is something that most healthcare professionals find distressing and difficult to cope with. Anger in a patient can escalate as he or she becomes irritated by more than one issue. Such anger can cause a healthcare team to lose confidence, and some professionals may react by using distancing tactics. Professionals may become defensive through a fear of litigation. An angry patient can cause distress both to their family and to other patients.

The healthcare professional should try to arrange for the consultation to be conducted in private in a quiet room without interruption. The anger needs to be acknowledged, and should not be dismissed as part of a coping process. The doctor needs to listen to the patient's story, eliciting all of their concerns. It is therapeutic for the patient to be allowed to vent their anger without interruption, facilitated by use of the principles of open questions and acknowledging the distress. The doctor should express feelings of sadness and regret at the situation without necessarily accepting the blame for it. 'Sorry' is possibly the most under-used word in these situations.

When helping the angry patient it is beneficial to explore feelings of guilt or depression associated with the anger. The professional may be tempted to dismiss the angry patient as uncooperative, but he should seek to understand the specific cause underlying such anger. The aggression can then be defused, allowing the patient to move towards acceptance.

If anger persists, it can be helpful for another team member such as a psychologist to talk to the patient to help them to recognise that no matter how justified the anger may be, it is affecting them adversely. Psychologists can also provide invaluable help by giving advice on simple anger management techniques, including relaxation or distraction activities.[5]

Denial

Case history

Mrs Brown is dying at home with advanced cancer of the ovary and sub-acute bowel obstruction. She is visited by her GP at home following discharge from hospital.

Doctor: 'Hello, Mrs Brown. How are you getting on after your recent stay in hospital?'
Mrs Brown: 'They were marvellous – I am sure I'm getting stronger.'

The initial reaction of patients on hearing bad news is often denial, and this should be accepted. It is important to check whether the patient wants to talk, as denial is an effective coping strategy which has been associated with prolonged survival in some studies.[6] The patient may give a strong signal that they do not wish to talk about their diagnosis or prognosis in a realistic way. Although research indicates that the majority of patients do want to be fully informed, it is important to respect the view of the small percentage who do not want to be given further information about their illness.[7]

A patient who denies their illness to one doctor may confide their fears to another member of staff. It may be that healthcare professionals who use denial as a coping strategy themselves encounter denial more frequently in their patients. Patients in denial are frightened, and they need patience and sensitive communication.

Not in front of the children

It is difficult to talk to children about death. Children are pragmatic and often demand information in a direct way. Older children have the same information needs as adults, but require it to be easily comprehended. Young children may need to assimilate information through the use of play, painting, videos and books. Like adults, children need to tell their story, and healthcare professionals need to be imaginative and uninhibited in helping them to articulate their distress. Parents often need support in breaking bad news to their children. An offer to help often involves sitting, listening and being with a family as they struggle to share bad news. Although specialist paediatric nurses, teachers, social workers and psychologists are very helpful, it will be the family doctor, health visitor or district nurse who is involved in the home. Generally the child will choose a favourite member of the professional team in whom they wish to confide. Children require and should receive the same ethical standards of honest information as adults.

Distancing tactics

Faced with the challenges discussed above, it is not surprising that healthcare professionals commonly adopt distancing tactics in an effort to avoid some of the stress of caring.[2]

Distancing tactics include physical avoidance, inappropriate reassurance or cheerfulness, ignoring cues, talking to patients following an examination while they are still undressed, and the use of jargon.

Physical avoidance

Extreme forms of distancing tactics result in avoidance of the patient. More subtle variations include talking to the patient from behind a desk, standing at the end of the bed, or entering data into a computer in order to avoid eye contact.

Inappropriate reassurance or cheerfulness

False or premature reassurance can prevent the patient from disclosing their concerns.

Ignoring cues

This is another way of maintaining distance. Generally patients will test whether the doctor is someone they can trust. If their cues are ignored, patients will quickly give up trying once they sense that the doctor is uncomfortable discussing their concerns in this area.[2] A doctor may miss a cue and distance himself, for example, by focusing on the physical elements of the problem and ignoring possible psychosexual problems. When a patient raises a difficult issue, it may be tempting to pass the problem on to a colleague and fail to respond to the patient's request for help.

Talking to patients following an examination while they are still undressed

Patients who are undressed are vulnerable and may be anxious and embarrassed. In this undignified state they will be unable either to assimilate any information or to participate in discussion.

Use of jargon

The use of medical terminology can distance the professional yet allow them to feel that they have been truthful.

Conclusion

Healthcare professionals should respond to the different information needs of the patient in an appropriate way. Communication is a dynamic process – it is not enough to record dispassionately 'patient is aware of diagnosis'. The level of understanding and progress of the patient must be reviewed regularly.

There are many challenges for healthcare professionals in their desire to communicate effectively, and an awareness of difficulties can improve practice. The empathy between the doctor and the patient is at the heart of good practice.

Key points

Honest communication lies at the heart of palliative care, and involves:

- concern and support for the patient and their family
- information about the illness and about treatment options
- commitment to do the best that can be done to relieve suffering
- respect for the patient's individuality and involvement in decision making
- availability and continuity of care
- awareness that healthcare professionals may adopt distancing tactics which block effective communication and avoid addressing the patient's real concerns.

References

1 Kaye P (1996) *Breaking Bad News: a ten-step approach*. EPL Publications, Northampton.
2 Faulkner A and Maguire P (1994) *Talking to Cancer Patients and Their Relatives*. Oxford University Press, Oxford.
3 National Cancer Alliance (1996) *Patient-Centred Cancer Services. What patients say*. National Cancer Alliance, Oxford.
4 Howie JGR, Heaney DJ, Maxwell M *et al*. (1999) Quality at general practice consultations: cross-sectional survey. *BMJ*. 319: 738–43.
5 Jeffrey D and Owen R (2003) Changing the emphasis from active curative care to active palliative care in haematology patients. In: S Booth and E Bruera (eds) *Palliative Care Consultations: haemato-oncology*. Oxford University Press, Oxford.

6 Greer S (1983) Cancer and the mind. *Br J Psychiatry*. **143**: 535–43.
7 Meredith C, Symonds P, Webster L *et al*. (1996) Information needs of cancer patients in west Scotland: cross-sectional survey of patients' views. *BMJ*. **313**: 724–6.

Part 2

Death, dying and dilemmas

6 'Am I going to die?': When cancer comes back

Out, out brief candle!
Life's but a walking shadow, a poor player
That struts and frets his hour upon the stage,
And then is heard no more.

Macbeth, V, v.

Case history

Jim, a 42-year-old teacher, developed bowel cancer two years ago. Following surgery and chemotherapy, he returned to work. He attends the oncology outpatient clinic for routine follow-up with his wife Jackie. During a clinical examination, the registrar finds that he has ascites and a hard enlarged liver.

The registrar returns from the examination room to the consulting room where Jackie is waiting. 'Is everything OK?', Jackie asks. Before the doctor can answer, Jim returns and, glancing at him, guesses that the news is bad.

Jim says to the doctor 'You look very serious – am I going to die?'. Jackie breaks down in tears.

The registrar faces several difficulties:

- supporting two distressed people
- possibly aggravating their distress
- feeling inadequate with regard to meeting their differing needs
- uncertainty as to how much he should tell the patient of his clinical impression that the cancer has recurred
- wanting to ask the consultant for advice
- there are 12 patients waiting in the clinic to see him.

Communication problems when cancer recurs

Giving news that a cancer has recurred or spread is difficult for doctors. This news may be harder for the patient and relatives to bear than the original diagnosis.

Breaking bad news

Breaking bad news is a process, not a single event. The doctor should respond to the needs of the individual patient rather than following any rigid protocol. However, Kaye's Ten Steps (*see* Box 6.1) provide a useful framework which can help professionals to cope with uncertain situations.[1] While the content of any communication should be honest and accurate, the manner of the communication is also important. The phrases used in the following paragraphs are intended only as illustrations to guide practice.

Box 6.1 Kaye's Ten Steps to Breaking Bad News[1]

1   Preparation
2   What does the patient know?
3   Is more information wanted?
4   Give a warning shot
5   Allow denial
6   Explain
7   Listen to concerns
8   Encourage ventilation of feelings
9   Summary and plan
10 Offer availability

Preparation

In the case described above, the doctor was surprised by the question '*Am I going to die?*'

It is important to ensure privacy, to establish whom the patient wishes to be present and to allow time for discussion. The healthcare professional should be familiar with the clinical information, including test results. Skilful preparation should include a plan to support the patient after the consultation. Is there another healthcare professional, such as a specialist nurse, who might be available to help?

What does the patient know?

It is risky to assume anything about the patient's understanding without first checking this out:

> 'Before we discuss the results of tests or treatment options, it would help me a great deal to know how much you understand about what is going on.'

In the above case the doctor might begin by acknowledging the distress:

> 'This is a difficult situation for you both. Please sit down, I need to take some time to address your concerns … Jim, before we talk about the future, could you tell me more about how you have been feeling?'

Jim may suspect that the cancer has returned, or he could have no idea that anything was wrong. Listening is essential to understanding the patient's view, and it gives the patient control.

Is more information wanted?

Most patients want to be fully informed, but it is helpful to check this:

> 'I have the results of the tests. Would you like me to explain, or are you the kind of person who doesn't want the medical details?'

Give a warning shot

Attending an oncology clinic is a 'warning shot' in itself, and in the case described above the doctor's worried expression alerted the patient. Another way of preparing a patient for bad news might be to say:

> 'I have some serious news that we will need to discuss.'

The warning, in whatever form, allows the patient to prepare psychologically to hear the bad news. It also gives them an opportunity to ask for a relative or friend to be present if they wish.

Allow denial

Patients are often frightened and shocked initially, and denial is an effective coping mechanism. The doctor needs to follow the patient's agenda and give information at the right pace to suit the individual patient.

If at a later date denial is causing difficulties – for instance, in discussing treatment options or addressing social problems – then it may be gently challenged:

'How do you feel things are going?'
'Do you ever think that it might be more serious?'

Explain

The information should be provided in simple non-technical language. The amount of information given needs to be matched to the patient's wishes.

Registrar: 'After my clinical examination I am concerned that your liver has become enlarged.'
Patient: 'Is it the cancer?'
Registrar: 'Although further tests will be needed to confirm it, I am sorry to say that it almost certainly means that the cancer has spread to your liver.'

Listen for concerns

The patient will usually want to discuss the implications of the bad news.

'Am I going to die?' is a difficult question that requires exploration in order to elicit the patient's specific concerns. Some patients worry that they may die within a few days, while others are more concerned about the manner of dying or about being a burden to others.

'That is a difficult question which I will do my best to answer, but before we discuss that can you tell me a little more about your concerns? What makes you ask about dying?'

There are many ways of screening for the patient's concerns. Non-verbal expressions of concern or silence can be powerful ways of eliciting the patient's view.

Other useful phrases might include the following:

> 'Please take your time. You have told me of your worries about how your wife will cope. Do you have any other concerns?'
>
> 'To be able to help you best, I need to understand – what are your concerns for the future?'

Encourage ventilation of feelings

Silence and touch may be appropriate to allow expression of emotions. Words that might help the patient to express their feelings include the following:

> 'I can see that this information is not what you expected.'
>
> 'Take your time, there's no need to apologise, it's OK to cry.'
>
> 'Your world seems to have turned upside down in such a short time ... it must be very difficult ...'
>
> 'There seem to be lots of things going wrong for you. Can you tell me what you feel is the worst thing about the situation?'

Often the doctor will feel intuitively that the patient is sad, angry or depressed:

> 'It seems to me that you are feeling angry ... could you tell me more about this please?'

Summary and plan

The doctor should identify one or two key points and check that the patient and relatives have understood. This can give the patient a chance to clarify their understanding of the treatment plan.

Offer availability

Continuity is one of the hallmarks of good palliative care. The patient will need further explanation of and information about available support. Other members of the team, including the general practitioner or specialist nurses, may play a vital role in supporting the patient.

Information can be supplied in written form, and some doctors record consultations concerning bad news on audiotape.

The patient and their relatives

The way in which the bad news is broken can influence a patient's subsequent adjustment to the illness and treatment.[2] The patient may have no suspicion that their situation is serious and may believe that their cancer has been cured. Such unrealistic hopes can be raised by over-optimistic doctors. For example, after the initial surgery the patient may be told that 'everything has been taken away'. Although an over-optimistic view may provide short-term reassurance, it will make the situation harder for the patient in the longer term, when the disease recurs. Healthcare professionals need to be cautious about using the term 'cure' in the context of most solid cancers in adults. 'Cure' may mean different things to the professional and the patient.

The patient and their family may have many concerns.[3]

- How long have I got? Fear for the future.
- Why me? The search for meaning.
- Am I still lovable? Body image and sexual concerns.
- What can I do? Fear of loss of control.
- Why won't they talk to me? Need for honesty.
- Will I be a burden to others? Fear of becoming dependent.
- Where is the doctor? Need for medical support.

Patients may have differing emotional reactions to the bad news, including shock, fear, anger, acceptance, sadness and resignation. Adjustment to bad news takes a variable amount of time. Initially denial is a common coping mechanism, acting as a psychological buffer against unexpected shocking news, and giving the patient time to prepare him- or herself. Each individual's reaction to hearing bad news varies, as there are no fixed steps to acceptance – the process is dynamic.

The patient's desire for information may change from day to day, as will their desire to participate in decision making.[4] Although the majority of patients wish to be fully informed, there is an important minority who have no wish to know their diagnosis. These patients usually make it very clear to their doctors that this is their way of coping. Such a choice should be respected so long as the doctor remembers that the patient is free to change their mind later and gives them the opportunity to do so. It is a mistake to label a patient as someone 'who wants to know' or 'who does not want to know'.

The doctor

The case described above illustrates some of the problems facing doctors who may experience strong emotions when they communicate bad news to a patient. If the patient displays emotions, as bearer of the bad news the doctor may feel that they are to blame in some way.

Alternatively, they may worry about displaying their emotions and feel that this is 'unprofessional'. Some doctors may feel that they have a duty to protect patients from the distress of hearing the bad news, fearing that the patient will give up hope if they become aware of the gravity of their situation. However, knowing a poor prognosis removes uncertainty, making many patients feel more secure. Hope is based on knowledge, whereas uncertainty leads to feelings of isolation.[5] Stress can interfere with a doctor's ability to communicate well. Thus taking a short break after a difficult consultation can enhance a doctor's effectiveness.[2] Training in communication skills for doctors is needed, and there is evidence that it can be effective.[6]

Ethical issues

Communication would become meaningless if there was no overriding moral obligation to be truthful. Honesty is an essential part of any trusting relationship. Patients with cancer need honest information to enable them to plan for the future. The question arises as to whether lying to patients can ever be justified. From a Kantian perspective there is a duty to tell the truth, and no blame can be attached to the doctor who tells the truth, even though this causes distress to the patient.[7] However, this rigid position is difficult to reconcile with the realities of clinical practice. The consequences of both truth telling and lying also need to be taken into consideration.

Morally there is little difference between an act (lying) and an omission (withholding the truth). In both situations there is a failure to fulfil the expectations of the doctor–patient relationship. The burden for justification must be on the doctor who wishes to lie or to withhold information from the patient. It is not only the individual act of lying which is morally relevant, but also the cumulative effect of such acts, which may lead to a public distrust of the medical profession. It is in their willingness to inform that a doctor demonstrates their respect for the patient's autonomy. Lying is a denial of autonomy, but could be justified by a paternalistic doctor either to prevent harm to the patient or to bring about a good. For instance, in the case described above, the doctor might withhold news of recurrent cancer from the patient, and instead arrange investigations in order to spare the patient distress and to confirm the doctor's clinical suspicions.

Doctors may be less than totally honest by arguing that the truth is not known. However, even if uncertainty exists, as in the case described above, this level of knowledge can be communicated to the patient in an honest and sensitive way. Uncertainty about the diagnosis, treatment or prognosis is no justification for lying. Doctors may also withhold information by using medical jargon that obscures the truth from the patient, or they may not feel obliged to tell 'the whole truth' even if the patient asks. Pressure of work may encourage conspiracies of silence rather than open discussion, as such discussion is time consuming. Doctors should not make assumptions about patients' needs, but rather they should base their communication on the patient's preferences.[4]

Challenging communications

Breaking bad news by telephone

If at all possible it is best to avoid giving bad news over the telephone. In rare instances doctors may have to discuss unexpected results of investigations over the telephone. Lee and colleagues have suggested the following guidelines which supplement the basic framework described above.[2]

- Acknowledge the difficulty of having to hold the discussion over the phone.
- Establish that the patient wants and is able to have a serious conversation.
- Find out whether the patient has support available.
- Do not give too many specific details.
- Try to find out how the patient is reacting.
- Arrange a follow-up appointment as soon as possible for the patient and their relatives.

Discussing the prognosis

Patients and their families need information in order both to gain a sense of control and to make plans. Relatives often want to know what is going to happen, and they may wish to be present at the death. Doctors are aware of the difficulties inherent in trying to estimate a prognosis for an individual. Information about the likely prognosis is indispensable for the doctor in determining whether to continue active treatments that have the potential for harm.

The patient may ask *'How long have I got?'*, in which case the doctor faces a number of problems.

- It is impossible to be certain what will happen to an individual.
- Doctors are often incorrect in their estimates of survival time.
- The doctor may fear distressing the patient.

By tailoring the Ten-Step framework discussed above to the needs of each individual, the doctor can try to understand what lies behind this question and what the patient really wants to know.

Acknowledging that it is a difficult question but one which can be explored forms a basis for gaining an understanding of the patient's concerns:

'That is an important but difficult question. I will do my best to answer you, but first we need to discuss the issue in a little more detail.'

It is important to gain some idea of the patient's view of the prognosis at an early stage:

'Before we go into more detail, I would find it very helpful if you could tell me what you think about your life expectancy.'

Some patients when told that the cancer has recurred fear they might die within a day or two, while others have high expectations of surviving a decade.

The doctor needs to try to find out what specific concerns the patient may have:

Doctor: 'The question you raise is clearly important. Can you tell me what particular issues in the future concern you?'
Patient: 'The real problem is that I must survive until my daughter's wedding in six months' time.'

There needs to be a discussion about the difficulties of predicting the future for an individual. It may be helpful to talk about the advantages and disadvantages that would exist if accurate knowledge was possible:

'If I was able, in some way, to be able to say exactly when you were going to die, are you sure that you would really want to know?'

The patient then has an opportunity to reflect on the implications for their quality of life of knowing exactly when it might end:

> 'Although it is well proven that doctors tend to be poor at estimating how long a patient may live, if you accept that, I can try to give a general idea. Would that be helpful?'

Some patients might find a best-case and worst-case scenario helpful:

> 'Some patients in a similar situation to you might survive two years, while others may become ill more quickly and only live for a few months.'

Statistics are generally confusing, and they rarely clarify the situation for patients. Both overestimating and underestimating survival time can cause distress. If the patient dies more quickly than predicted he may be left with unfinished business, and if he survives longer than the prognosis, the relatives may have become physically and mentally exhausted.

Some patients deal best with a limited prognosis by setting realistic goals:

> 'What is the next goal that you have? Have you any things that you are looking forward to doing in the next few weeks?'
> 'Once you have enjoyed your holiday in a month's time you might find it helpful to set another goal.'

Sometimes these discussions may involve a lowering of the patient's expectations:

> 'Until we see how your cancer will progress, perhaps it would be better to set some goals which you would like to achieve in the next few months, rather than looking at what might happen in two years' time.'

The discussion may include talking about the patient's fears of death and dying:

> 'Would you like to talk a little more about your fears for the future?'
> 'Some patients with cancer worry a great deal about how it will be for them when they come to the end of their life. Do you have any fears that you would like to talk about?'

Communication strategies can be helpful, but the healthcare professional needs to remember that there is no one right way. Rather they should adopt an open approach that allows them to share their vulnerability as well as their expertise with the patient.

Collusion

Doctor–relative collusion

Case history

Charles, a 50-year-old farmer, was diagnosed with a gastric carcinoma. His wife approached the surgeon and asked him not to tell her husband about the severity of his condition: 'Please don't tell him – he's not used to illness and would just give up.'

The surgeon faces a number of problems.

- He has a duty to inform the patient.
- He does not want to breach confidentiality.
- He does not want to distress the patient's wife further.
- He wants to continue to have her trust and help with the future care of the patient.

Most doctors will have experienced a request from a relative to conceal information from the patient. In such cases there is clearly a conflict between the doctor's duty to the patient and his responsibility to care for and support the family.

The key to promoting openness is to recognise that the request 'please don't tell him' is a cry for help. The first task is to gain permission from the patient to speak to his wife on her own:

'Your wife is obviously concerned about you. Are you happy for me to talk to her about your condition, on her own, to try to help her?'

When talking to the patient's wife it is important to establish what she thinks the patient knows, and her understanding of the disease:

'I can see that you are very concerned for your husband. You know him best – could you tell me what you think he understands of his condition?'

During this consultation the surgeon can check the wife's understanding and explore her reasons for not telling her husband:

'What is your understanding of your husband's disease?'
'Can you tell me why you feel it is so important that he should not be told that he has stomach cancer?'

Relatives may also not have appreciated that the consequence of collusion is greater isolation from the patient. Furthermore, maintaining such a deception is stressful:

'What effects have your husband's illness had on you? It must be difficult for you at times.'

In the case described above, once the patient's wife can see that the doctor is sensitive to her husband's best interests, she may well 'allow' him to explore her husband's understanding and to give him the information that he needs. It is often helpful to suggest that the patient has almost certainly guessed what is wrong.

This supportive approach is time consuming, but it saves a great deal of family distress in the long term. Statements like '*He is my patient – I have to tell him*' may be technically correct, but would do nothing to address the wife's distress in the above case.

Doctor–patient collusion

Case history[8]

Henry and his wife have come to see the consultant for the results of a chest X-ray.

Doctor: 'Unfortunately, the tests show that it is lung cancer.'

The consultant pauses.

Henry: 'How long have I got, doctor?'
Doctor: 'This type of lung cancer is aggressive – it grows fast. On the other hand, it is very sensitive to chemotherapy. It certainly can be treated.'

> The consultant continues to explain the nature and side-effects of chemotherapy.
>
> Henry (interrupting):   'I want to try everything.'
> Doctor: 'I'll try to arrange that you can start chemotherapy tomorrow.'

In one study, almost all patients with small-cell lung cancer who were receiving chemotherapy were found to have a 'false optimism' about their recovery.[8] This is significant, because the patient's ideas about their prognosis may influence their treatment choices.

In this study, details of the likely progress of the disease and the prognosis were rarely given. Patients were told that it is difficult to give a prognosis because each individual is unique. In most cases this statement was followed by an offer of chemotherapy. Most of the time was spent talking about treatment options – the patient and the doctor colluded in discussing these rather than the prognosis and disease progression.[8]

The patient's reluctance to ask about the prognosis was interpreted by doctors as 'not wanting to know'. The and her colleagues found that doctors used ambiguous words in consultations – for example, 'your lungs are clear' or 'treatment is possible' – which had positive implications.[8] Even when doctors stated that the treatment was palliative, patients persisted in believing that there was a chance of cure. This pretence that recovery was possible was maintained into the terminal stages of the disease. False optimism hampered patients in preparing for death, and this was a cause for regret when these patients and their families eventually realised that death was imminent.

Awareness of a poor prognosis can be facilitated by good communication skills and attention to non-verbal cues. Professionals need to enable patients to assimilate bad news rather than hastily offering them treatments, which patients tend to seize upon when in a state of shock.

As the illness progresses, doctors may be tempted to focus on the treatment plan, giving the patient no chance to reflect on their limited lifespan. The collusion continues as patients also tend to feel secure and valued in an environment of medical activity. However, The's research highlights the fact that, in the longer term, not only patients but also their relatives regret the missed opportunity to complete unfinished emotional business. They conclude that 'it is not in the patient's interest to adhere to the "treatment calendar" in the early phases of the illness trajectory'.[8]

Cultural influences

Doctors should be aware of the variety of different cultural attitudes to death. However, they should not make assumptions when talking to an individual from an ethic minority. It is best to address possible cross-cultural differences quite openly with the patient.[2] There is a need to distinguish between cultural diversity and fundamental ethical principles. Respect for autonomy, which is a fundamental ethical principle, includes respect for the values of the individual patient. Individuals' values often reflect those of their culture, but they do not always do so.[9]

Emotional responses

A patient may react with anger on receiving bad news. When confronted by such a response, the doctor may be tempted to dismiss this as the patient's problem. However, the doctor should recognise that he himself is suffering similar emotions of frustration. An awareness that these strong feelings are shared by both doctor and patient enables the doctor to empathise with the patient rather than aggravating their distress.[2]

Depression

Depression may be difficult to diagnose in patients with advanced cancer. The symptoms can range from the patient being suicidal to a more subtle situation in which the patient may not acknowledge depression. Surprisingly, it is sometimes a doctor's feelings of sadness that may point to depression in the patient.[2]

When assessing depression a direct approach is most effective: '*Do you sometimes feel depressed?*' Some patients may be reluctant to talk, so the healthcare professional should show a readiness to listen to the patient's feelings.

A range of assessment measures of depression is available.[10]

Improving communication

Communication with patients and colleagues can be improved by understanding the reasons for communication breakdown. The challenge for healthcare professionals is to tailor information to meet the individual patient's changing needs and preferences.

Communication skills that help to elicit the patient's concerns and enable them to talk openly about their feelings, thereby establishing empathy, include the following:[11]

- the use of open questions
- maintaining appropriate eye contact
- asking about the patient's worries and feelings
- clarifying psychological issues
- summarising the discussion.

Can communication skills be acquired?

Fallowfield and colleagues have conducted communication skills training workshops which were evaluated by means of videos. They demonstrated that after the workshops the doctors used more expressions of empathy, more often responded appropriately to patients' cues and used fewer leading questions.[6] The skills learned in training workshops need to be used and practised in a clinical setting. Good communication skills require reinforcement through further training, feedback and support from colleagues.[12]

Key points

- Communicating bad news is a core clinical skill.
- Patients cannot express preferences about their care unless they are given appropriate information.
- The great majority of cancer patients want honest information about their illness.
- The manner of the communication as well as its content is of ethical importance.
- Healthcare professionals need to elicit the patient's needs and readiness for information.
- Training and support can improve the communication skills of healthcare professionals.

References

1 Kaye P (1996) *Breaking Bad News: a ten-step approach*. EPL Publications, North-ampton.
2 Lee SJ, Back AL, Block SD *et al.* (2002) Enhancing physician–patient communication. *Haematology*. **1:** 464.
3 Faulkner A and Maguire P (1994) *Talking to Cancer Patients and Their Relatives*. Oxford University Press, Oxford.
4 Fallowfield L (2003) Communication with the patient and family in palliative medicine. In: D Doyle *et al.* (eds) *Oxford Textbook of Palliative Medicine* (3e). Oxford University Press, Oxford.
5 Fallowfield L, Jenkins VA and Beveridge HA (2002) Truth may hurt but deceit hurts more: communication in palliative care. *Palliat Med*. **16:** 297–303.
6 Fallowfield L, Jenkins V, Fovewell V *et al.* (2002) Efficacy of a Cancer Research UK communication skills model: a randomised controlled trial. *Lancet*. **359:** 650–6.
7 Palmer M (1999) *Moral Problems in Medicine*. Lutterworth Press, Cambridge.
8 The A-M, Hak T, Koeter G *et al.* (2000) Collusion in doctor–patient communication about imminent death: an ethnographic study. *BMJ*. **321:** 1376–81.
9 Macklin R (1999) *Against Relativism*. Oxford University Press, Oxford.
10 Lloyd-Williams M and Friedman T (2001) Depression in palliative care patients – a prospective study. *Eur J Cancer Care*. **10:** 270–74.
11 Heaven C and Maguire P (1998) The relationship between patients' concerns and psychological distress in a hospice setting. *Psycho-oncology*. **7:** 502–7.
12 Wilkinson S, Roberts A and Aldridge J (1998) Nurse–patient communication in palliative care: an evaluation of a communication skills programme. *Palliat Med*. **14:** 308–12.

7 'What should I do?': Informed consent

O, but they say the tongues of dying men
Enforce attention like deep harmony:
Where words are scarce, they are seldom spent in vain;
For they breathe truth that breathe their words in pain.

King Richard II, II, i.

Case history

Charles Wood, a 50-year-old forester, lives with his wife Margaret. He is a lifelong smoker and has recently been investigated for a persistent cough and breathlessness. He attends the outpatient clinic to find out the results of investigations performed ten days earlier. He is shown into the office of Dr Grainger, a chest physician, whose clinic is running an hour and a half behind schedule.

Dr Grainger (*standing next to an X-ray viewing box showing a chest X-ray*): 'Hello, Mr Wood, have you come on your own today?'
Charles: 'No. Margaret, my wife, is waiting outside.'
Dr Grainger: 'Would you like her to come in?'
Charles: 'I'd like to hear the results of my tests first.'
Dr Grainger (*sitting down and looking down at the case notes*): 'I'm afraid the news is not good.'
Charles: 'Is it cancer?'
Dr Grainger (*looking up at the patient and appearing sad*): 'Well, yes, I'm sorry to say that it is ... it's a type of cancer of the lung.'
Charles: 'Is there any treatment?'
Dr Grainger (*looking much brighter and sounding positive*): 'Oh yes, although with this sort of cancer surgery is not very helpful. I think

that it could respond well to drugs – treatment called chemotherapy. I think that you might well benefit from chemotherapy.'

Charles: 'Thank God for that. Margaret's sister had chemo for cancer some years ago and she is really well. Will I have to come into hospital straightaway?'

Dr Grainger *(glancing momentarily at his watch)*: 'I will need to refer you to an oncologist who will tell you more about chemotherapy. You will get a letter from Dr Green, the oncologist who will see you shortly.'

Background

Gillon has defined informed consent as follows:

> A voluntary uncoerced decision, made by a sufficiently competent or autonomous person, on the basis of adequate information and deliberation to accept rather than reject some proposed course of action that will affect him or her.[1]

Patients have a right to make informed decisions about their care, a right which is protected in law.[2] Informed consent is an important mechanism for protecting patients from medical paternalism. The Bristol Inquiry stated 'We believe that healthcare professionals have a duty to empower patients. Providing information is one means of empowerment'.[3] The notion of consent emphasises the duty of the doctor to give information about the risks of any proposed intervention.[4]

A voluntary decision

A patient should be able to choose or reject a proposed treatment freely, without coercion or deception. In seeking informed consent, the distinction between coercion and persuasion may be lost. Persuasion aims to enlist the patient's cooperation by providing information, but coercion manipulates a patient's decision by undermining their independent reasoning. In the case described above the doctor swiftly accepted the patient's decision, even though it was made immediately after hearing the news that he had cancer. After waiting a long time to see the consultant, the patient may feel under pressure not to take more of his time – this is a form of coercion. The patient in the above case was referred to an oncologist without being given time to discuss this option with his family. Another way in which unethical coercion may influence decisions is by implying that a patient will be discharged without further treatment if he does not take the doctor's advice. Alternatively, the patient may be given insufficient information and be coerced into a course of treatment without fully understanding the implications of this.

The doctor in the case described above also failed to clarify what type of cancer the patient's sister-in-law suffered, nor did he challenge the patient's optimistic expectations of chemotherapy. From the moment of diagnosis a form of collusion developed between the doctor and the patient. The doctor's perceived level of concern can also influence the patient's perception of how much he or she is being informed.

A sufficiently competent person

A doctor who is concerned with informing a patient needs to assess the patient's competence to make autonomous decisions. The doctor must first assess the patient's ability to understand, as this is central to the concept of consent.[5] Competence with regard to understanding a treatment or research trial involves the patient's ability to weigh risks against benefits and to make a choice based on this understanding. A patient is competent if he or she can comprehend information when it has been clearly presented, and retain it long enough to weigh it up and make a decision.[2]

The assessment of a patient's decision-making capacity is an integral part of the communication between doctor and patient. However, *competence* is also a legal concept that covers the skill of communicating, understanding and retaining the relevant information and using it rationally to make a choice. The Adults with Incapacity (Scotland) Act 2000 and the Mental Capacity Bill are frameworks for substitute decision making for people who are unable to make decisions for themselves. The Mental Capacity Bill makes provision for those with full capacity to draw up 'lasting powers of attorney' to take health decisions on their behalf should they later become incapacitated. The proxy will be able to refuse or consent to medical treatment if the patient has authorised it. In addition, the Mental Capacity Bill has provision on advance directives which allows patients to specify, while still capable, what treatment they want to refuse in the event of their later losing capacity.[6]

If a patient does not fully comprehend the information that is given to him or her, further explanation must be given before seeking consent. This also applies to patients who have capacity but who cannot understand the information because of problems with literacy or language.[5]

Some patients are obviously incompetent to make decisions (e.g. when unconscious), but there are many cases where the situation is not so clear-cut. In the case described above, the patient may have been shocked by the bad news and be judged to be temporarily incompetent to make a decision about his future treatment. Patients with cancer may also have fluctuating levels of confusion due to biochemical changes associated with advanced disease.

Depending on the urgency of the situation, the doctor may wait until the patient's condition has improved or they may, in an emergency, make a decision which is in their judgement in the 'best interests' of the patient. In these situations the doctor is acting paternalistically. Great care must be taken to review the patient and to avoid misinterpreting different cultural ideas about illness as indicating a lack of comprehension. If the patient can become capable of a level of understanding that is adequate to enable them to make autonomous choices, the case for paternalistic intervention is weak. However, below this level of competence the case for paternalism is stronger, and the duty of beneficence assumes a greater priority than that of autonomy.

In determining the patient's best interests the doctor needs to consider three factors, namely the options for treatment which are clinically indicated, any previously expressed wishes of the patient, and any relevant cultural or religious issues. Any views about the patient's wishes given by a third party, family member or tutor-dative (in Scotland) will be relevant. The doctor should also seek the option that least restricts the patient's future choices.[2]

A sufficiently autonomous person

A central component of a life worth living is respect for autonomy, which is protected by a requirement for informed and understood consent. Informed consent, like 'breaking bad news', is a process whereby the patient and the healthcare professional come to a clear understanding. An informed choice gives the patient a sense of being in control, making choices consciously and recognising a degree of uncertainty. The satisfaction derived from exercising one's autonomy may be more important than making the choice with the highest expected value. Patients do not necessarily make conservative decisions when they are fully informed about the risks and benefits of treatment options.

Moody has argued that formal mechanisms of informed consent may be inadequate for protecting a patient's autonomy. He makes a plea for a concept which he calls 'negotiated consent', which involves shared decision making between the patient, the family and the professionals.[7] Similarly, Towle and Godolphin extend the concept of informed consent to 'informed shared decision making'.[8] In both articles the authors are emphasising the importance of a patient-centred approach to informed consent.

Adequate information and deliberation

A patient-centred approach concentrates on the need for full information, setting limits on the doctor's perception and beliefs. Doctors may have an undue influence on patients' decisions, and a clear presentation of facts is only possible if the doctor is circumspect about his or her own fears and beliefs. However, the patient should not be manipulated into having to make choices in isolation if the doctor is uncertain or does not discuss treatment options.

A patient-centred approach encourages doctors to understand the patient's fears and values. Doctors need to discuss risk in terms other than survival statistics when offering treatment options. Patients need an opportunity to ask questions about what they have been told, and should be free to ask for more information if they wish.[5]

The legal requirements with regard to what information needs to be given to the patient for proper consent are evolving in case law.[9] Under the Bolam test, the professional standard by which disclosure to patients is judged is that which would be endorsed by a reasonable body of medical opinion.[10] However, in the Bolitho case the House of Lords determined that an unreasonable failure to disclose may now render a clinician liable in damages, whatever his colleagues declare to be reasonable practice.[11] This 'reasonable person standard' is based on whether a reasonable person in that patient's position would wish to be informed.[4] The courts have ruled that the ultimate legal test is what the court considers was a reasonable amount of information to give the patient.[9] This leaves the doctor in the predicament of having to guess the decision of the court.

Patients may want a variety of information before consenting to treatment, including details of the diagnosis and prognosis, levels of uncertainty and risk, treatment options, common and serious side-effects and the likely benefits, with probabilities of success.[2] Often there is no formula that can tell a doctor which treatment option is 'best' for an individual patient. Doctors should offer alternatives and discuss treatment choices. This sharing option is clinically and emotionally more demanding for doctors, and requires sensitivity to the changing needs of the patient.

Although the patient and the doctor may share a common understanding initially, as time passes and the cancer progresses, patients and physicians may develop divergent views on the aims of the therapy. Patients in a palliative setting who are receiving treatment that is directed at relieving symptoms may well believe that the therapy is aimed at disease control.

The attitude of the healthcare professional is a key factor in determining whether the patient is informed and what choice he or she makes.

The needs of the patient are the main priority, but the views of relatives should also be considered, although a relative cannot give consent in place of an adult patient. If there is a conflict between these views, time needs to be spent exploring the reasons for the differences and giving people time to adjust to new situations.

Case history

Charles Wood sees the oncologist, Dr Green, who explains that his lung cancer has a good chance of responding to a course of chemotherapy.

Dr Green: 'This type of lung cancer is a serious form, but it has a good chance of responding to chemotherapy. The exact form of the combination of drugs will be determined by the research protocol in a randomised clinical trial. There are risks to the treatment which are uncommon, but some of which may be serious.'

Charles: 'I didn't realise that it was an experiment.'

Dr Green: 'Well, most new cancer drugs are used in large research trials ... if you are interested in having this treatment then the research nurse will see you and explain all the details.'

Charles: 'I don't really know – what should I do?'

The patient in the above case history may choose not to be informed fully, or to leave the decision to the professional. Such a waiver of informed consent does not mean that the patient is giving up his right to information in the future. However, the patient may just wish to be helpful, and part of a doctor's skill is to see beyond the brave face and to explore the real wishes of the patient. The doctor needs to be certain that the patient is not being driven by a wish to be helpful.

For doctors and patients to face uncertainty together there must be trust between them. A framework for informed consent enables patients to make their own decisions by considering their own probabilities and values as a basis for making a decision. The patient, the relatives and the healthcare professionals need to weigh the burdens of the treatment against the realistic benefits.

Communication and consent

A communication spectrum exists, ranging from the patient demanding a futile treatment at one extreme, to the doctor acting as an advocate of the patient, empowering them to make their own choices, to the doctor making the decision for the patient at the other extreme (*see* Box 7.1). The role of the doctor in palliative care is as much informant, advocate and facilitator as it is diagnostician and decision maker.

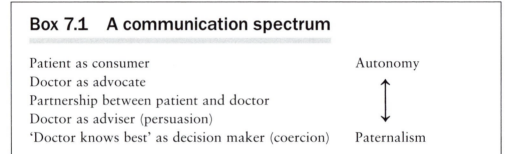

Box 7.1   A communication spectrum

Patient as consumer	Autonomy
Doctor as advocate	
Partnership between patient and doctor	
Doctor as adviser (persuasion)	
'Doctor knows best' as decision maker (coercion)	Paternalism

An ethical form of communication requires that the parties involved are given honest information, with an opportunity to negotiate and reflect on their choices.

The doctor's attitude and manner of communication are crucial in influencing the patient's choices. If the doctor feels a sense of failure and equates palliative care with giving up, then the patient will rapidly pick this up from non-verbal cues. Delegation of this vital explanation and discussion to nurses may be a pragmatic way of giving patients information. Doctors should ensure that the nurses have the necessary knowledge to answer the questions that may arise and offer follow-up support to their nursing colleagues.

Explaining risks and acknowledging uncertainty

Successful risk communication depends on establishing a relationship of mutual respect and trust between the doctor and the patient. Trust is a function of care and competence and is integral to credibility. Trust between doctor and patient fosters the process of communicating risk. Patients are enabled to persist with a decision for long enough to enable them to assess its long-term as well as immediate outcomes, and it gives them time to change their minds.

Professional virtues of competence, honest and empathy are all relevant in communicating risk – merely describing the facts in a way that can be understood is not enough. Doctors need to acknowledge uncertainty, and this may be uncomfortable for both patients and healthcare professionals.[12]

Improving communication in consent

Effective risk communication forms the basis for achieving informed patient consent, yet doctors are largely untrained in these skills.[13] The majority of patients with advanced cancer are in an anxious state when they see doctors, and their comprehension and recall skills are diminished. Such patients tend to extract a vague outline of any information that is given to them, rather than the detail, and tend to make an assessment of the risks based on emotions.[14,15]

Open and honest communication between staff and patients requires the doctor to display a competent and caring approach which fosters a trusting relationship. Paling has suggested a number of useful steps for communicating risk.[13]

- Empathise with the emotions of the patient.
- Avoid using descriptive terms alone (e.g. rather than just saying 'low risk', provide estimated numbers).
- Use a common denominator (e.g. 40 out of 1000 and 5 out of 1000 rather than 1 in 25 and 1 in 200). Some patients will think 1 in 200 is a bigger risk than 1 in 25.
- Offer positive and negative outcomes (e.g. chances of side-effects occurring and of remaining free from side-effects).
- Use absolute numbers, not relative risks.
- Use visual aids to describe probabilities.
- Ensure that all consent is 'informed'.
- Express encouragement and hope by describing the support available.

One of the challenges facing clinicians is how to interpret the results of clinical trials in a meaningful way for individual patients. It may be necessary to have translations, interpreters, signers or a patient's representative available to help in situations where communication is likely to be difficult. Sometimes the presence of a relative or friend may help, as may the tape recording of the consultation. Allowing time for reflection is imperative, and if the doctor's time is too limited then involving other members of the healthcare team is appropriate. Patients should be encouraged to question doctors and review their decisions, and to change their minds if they wish. The way in which doctors communicate risks affects the patient's perception of the risks of a proposed intervention.

Medical students are taught interviewing and history taking, but not much about giving patients information or communicating risk.[16] Doctors ought to be able to state options: 'You have some choices, and they are …'.[16] They need to discuss the options in the light of the patient's preferences, and to respond to the patient's ideas, concerns and expectations. Patients often find it difficult to question a doctor. They may feel intimidated, or that they are wasting time or may jeopardise rapport.[8]

Consent in medical research

Patients who are no longer curable by standard treatments are vulnerable to exposure to new therapies in clinical research trials. Alternatively, patients may demand an untested treatment that they have read or heard about in the media. Unless these treatments are subjected to research trials involving patients, doctors will lack the scientific evidence necessary to judge which of them are most effective. Thus there is a conflict between the doctor's duty to do the best for his individual patient and his responsibility to develop improved treatments for the future. Informed consent can be a valuable mechanism for moderating scientific progress to a pace that shows care and respect for patients. It ensures that the patient as the subject of therapeutic research is respected as an individual and not used as a means to others' ends. Such consent makes doctors more aware of the effects of their intervention and more accountable for their decisions. There is a need to help patients to distinguish the risks of clinical care from the additional risks of participating in a research trial.[4] Obtaining informed consent is therefore essential if doctors are to meet appropriate standards of clinical care and therapeutic research.

Obtaining such consent can be difficult in palliative care settings, particularly in dying patients. A process of advance consent has been proposed as one way of enabling the ethical recruitment to research trials of patients who are unable to give consent at the time of randomisation.[17]

Conclusions

All medical interventions – whether diagnostic, therapeutic or for research – have the potential to violate patient autonomy. The central function of informed consent is to ensure a sharing of power and knowledge between doctor and patient. Through this sharing process the patient receives appropriate care from doctors whom they trust, and doctors gain a deeper understanding of the patient's needs. Informed consent can be viewed as an expression of two elements of care – one responsive to the patient's wishes and the other protective against harmful intervention. Informed consent is a dialogue between a patient and their doctor in which both become aware of the potential harms and benefits for the patient. It is much more than a mere granting of permission.

Key points

- A patient should be able to choose or reject a proposed treatment freely without coercion.
- A doctor who is concerned with informing a patient needs to assess the patient's competence to make autonomous decisions.
- Informed consent, like breaking bad news, is a process.
- The attitude of the healthcare professional is a key factor in determining whether the patient is informed.
- For doctors and patients to face uncertainty together there must be trust between them.
- The role of the doctor in palliative care is as much informant, advocate and facilitator as it is diagnostician and decision maker.
- Informed consent can be a valuable mechanism for moderating scientific progress to a pace that shows care and respect for patients.
- Doctors require education in communicating risk.

References

1 Gillon R (1985) *Philosophical Medical Ethics*. John Wiley & Sons, Chichester.
2 General Medical Council (1998) *Seeking Patients' Consent: the ethical considerations*. General Medical Council, London.
3 Bristol Royal Infirmary Inquiry (2001) *The Inquiry into the Management of Care of*

Children Receiving Complex Heart Surgery at the Bristol Royal Infirmary. Command Paper 5207. Bristol Royal Infirmary Inquiry, Bristol.

4 Mazur DJ (2003) Influence of the law on risk and informed consent. *BMJ.* **327:** 731–6.

5 Mayberry MK and Mayberry JF (2002) Consent with understanding: a movement towards informed decisions. *Clin Med JRCPL.* **2:** 523–6.

6 Dyer C (2004) Living wills have to specify treatments that patient is refusing. *BMJ.* **328:** 1035.

7 Moody HR (1988) From informed consent to negotiated consent. *Gerontologist.* **28:** 64–70.

8 Towle A and Godolphin W (1999) Framework for teaching and learning informed shared decision making. *BMJ.* **319:** 766–71.

9 Smith AM (2001) Obtaining consent for examination and treatment. *BMJ.* **322:** 810–11.

10 *Bolam v Friern Hospital Management Committee* [1957] 1 WLR 582–94.

11 *Bolitho v City & Hackney Health Authority* [1998] AC 232.

12 Edwards A (2003) Communicating risks. *BMJ.* **327:** 691–2.

13 Paling J (2003) Strategies to help patients understand risks. *BMJ.* **327:** 745–8.

14 Lloyd A, Hayes P, Bell RF *et al.* (2001) The role of risk and benefit perception in informed consent for surgery. *BMJ.* **320:** 909–13.

15 Ropiek D and Clay G (2002) *Risk! A practical guide for deciding what's really safe and what's dangerous in the world around you.* Oxford University Press, Oxford.

16 Godolphin W (2003) *The Role of Risk Communication in Shared Decision Making.* Oxford University Press, Oxford.

17 Rees E and Hardy J (2003) Novel consent process for research in dying patients unable to give consent. *BMJ.* **327:** 198.

8 'What are you going to do next?': The limits of palliative chemotherapy

> I wasted time, and now doth time waste me.
> *King Richard II,* V, v.

Introduction

The withholding or withdrawal of chemotherapy needs to be examined if patients with advanced cancer are to receive appropriate care. The potential benefits and burdens of palliative chemotherapy should be weighed up carefully.[1] These are summarised in Table 8.1.

Table 8.1 Potential benefits and burdens of palliative chemotherapy

Advantages	Disadvantages
Symptom relief	Toxicity
Prolonged survival	Time lost to treatment
Reduced tumour size	Psychological morbidity
Improved activity	Social disruption
Hope of improvement	Death
Treatment plan	Fears of treatment
	Reminders of disease
	Loss of autonomy
	Uncertainty
	Role change

Aims of palliative chemotherapy

In the palliative phase of care, the most important consideration is the patient's quality of life. The aim of giving chemotherapy to patients with advanced cancer should be to optimise the patient's quality of life.[2] Assessment of their quality of life may be problematic, as measurement of the outcomes of chemotherapy which relate to the patient's priorities is difficult.

Many chemotherapy trials have no quality-of-life measures which reflect the patient's concerns, but rather are measures of health status. Patients who are recruited into research trials of palliative chemotherapy may be a fitter group with a better prognosis than those who are excluded from such trials. There is a risk that the results of a trial derived from these fitter patients will then be applied in the clinical setting to less fit patients who would have been rejected from the original trial.

Uncertainties exist for both patients and healthcare professionals with regard to the appropriate time to cease palliative chemotherapy. Clinicians may be in a dilemma as they seek to avoid over-treating patients on the one hand and neglecting a remote chance of prolonged survival on the other.[3]

Palliative chemotherapy is an intervention that involves the use of drugs to help to relieve pain or other distressing symptoms. The use of such therapy raises difficult questions, as there is no clear relationship between a reduction in size of the tumour and relief of symptoms. The role of palliative chemotherapy in treating an asymptomatic patient is controversial. Some forms of chemotherapy may be used with the intention of reducing tumour bulk and slowing the advance of the disease. However, if no symptoms are present, it is difficult to identify which patients will develop problems and are most likely to benefit from such chemotherapy.

If chemotherapy is being given with curative intent, prolongation of life is the commonest measure of success. In a palliative context the extension of life may be minimal, but some side-effects of chemotherapy are serious enough to result in death. Although some patients might be prepared to accept a risk of death if there was also the chance of cure, it seems unacceptable that a palliative treatment should carry a risk of death or serious side-effects. Patients need honest information on risks and benefits, because even a slim chance of a short prolongation of life may be important for some individuals.

Some patients and doctors may be using palliative chemotherapy treatment regimes as a way of avoiding confronting end-of-life issues and of raising false hopes. There is a feeling that chemotherapy may be overused at the end of life.[4]

Some palliative chemotherapy regimes may be part of research trials, raising questions about the ethics of research on dying patients. The problem of achieving informed and understood consent for such research must be addressed.

Death and dying may be perceived as failures of medical technology, rather than as an appropriate and natural consequence of advanced cancer. Patients or their families may try to persuade doctors to continue with chemotherapy regimes even when the doctor has suggested that they are no longer beneficial.

Doctors from different disciplines may interpret identical data from research trials of palliative chemotherapy in different ways. For example, a systematic review of the use of palliative chemotherapy for advanced colorectal cancer found that chemotherapy improved median survival by 3.7 months, but noted that the quality of evidence relating to treatment toxicity, symptom control and quality of life was poor.[5]

In any study designed to assess the value of palliative chemotherapy, it is vital to weigh the benefits of chemotherapy against treatment toxicity and the effect on the patient's quality of life. These issues were clearly not adequately addressed in the research reviewed on advanced colorectal cancer. Surprisingly, in the same journal in which that study was reported, an editorial concluded that 'there is now strong evidence to suggest that chemotherapy should be offered to all patients with advanced colorectal cancer, depending on their physical functioning'.[6]

Case history

Frank, a 74-year-old retired teacher, was diagnosed with cancer of the colon with liver metastases. He was offered palliative chemotherapy, but suffered from diarrhoea and had to be admitted to hospital, where investigations revealed that the cancer was progressing. The oncologist, Dr Swan, saw him on the ward round.

Dr Swan: 'Good morning, Frank. How are you feeling today?'
Frank: 'Much better, thank you. What are you going to treat me with next?'
Dr Swan: 'The chemotherapy seems to have made you feel much worse, and the results of your scan show that the drugs were not controlling the cancer.'
Frank: 'So what are you going to do now?'
Dr Swan: 'We could try a second-line type of chemotherapy, but I feel that you may not respond well to it. Also it could have worse side-

> effects than the first course. I would recommend that we should stop drug treatments and instead give you time to recover your strength and see my colleagues in the palliative care team.'
>
> Frank: 'So you are saying there is nothing more that anyone can do?'

Introducing palliative care

Just because an option for chemotherapy exists does not mean that it must be used. In some dying patients, doctors may persist with chemotherapy to avoid a sense of guilt about 'abandoning' the patient. They may fear that confronting the patient with the goals of palliative care will prove too distressing or will destroy all hope. The situation is complicated further if the patient or their family demand further treatment directed against the disease. In the midst of all this medical activity the patient may be denied access to specialist palliative care.

Communication

It may be difficult to communicate the news that active chemotherapy should cease. There is a lack of privacy on a ward round which may inhibit the patient from asking questions or expressing emotion. Pressure of time may result in a prescription rather than an exploration of the patient's concerns. The prognosis for an individual patient is often uncertain. Oncologists can always recall a particular patient who responded unexpectedly well to palliative chemotherapy, achieving a prolonged survival with good quality of life. It may be simpler to give way to these pressures and give futile active treatment rather than acknowledge the difficult situation with the patient and family. However, doctors are neither legally nor morally obliged to offer futile treatments. Giving chemotherapy as a way of maintaining hope does not seem to be an ethical use of scarce resources.

Collusion in doctor–patient communication

The's qualitative study of doctor–patient communication in 35 patients with lung cancer was discussed in Chapter 6.[7] 'False optimism about recovery' usually developed during the first course of chemotherapy, and was most prevalent when the cancer was no longer present on the chest X-ray. Patients slowly became aware of the poor prognosis through physical deterioration and as a result of contact with fellow patients with more advanced disease. In the outpatient clinic setting, patients rarely dealt with their approaching death. The identified five stages in a common disease trajectory:[7]

1   existential crisis at diagnosis
2   focus on treatment during the first chemotherapy course
3   relative peace of mind when the cancer was not visible on X-ray
4   existential crisis at the diagnosis of disease recurrence
5   final crisis when receiving news that there was no further effective treatment.

It was during the third of these stages that patients felt 'cured' and optimism was at its height. The fact that patients did not ask for further information caused the poor prognosis to be concealed. There was a rapid transition between giving the diagnosis and discussion of the treatment available, with most of the time being spent on 'treatment options'. Treatment was offered giving the patient a hope of cure, despite the doctor's explanation that the aims of therapy were palliative. A possible solution to this problem is not to force information on patients but to use 'treatment brokers' outside the close oncologist–patient relationship to help patients to come to terms with the reality of their situation.[7] Other studies have confirmed that patients did not understand the extent of their disease, and that their doctors often failed to recognise this lack of understanding.[8] Silvestri and colleagues studied patients with lung cancer who had been treated, and showed that patients varied widely in their willingness to accept chemotherapy for metastatic lung cancer. Many would not choose chemotherapy for its likely survival benefit of three months, but would choose it if it improved their quality of life.[9] It is of concern that the study revealed some patients had not received the treatment they would have chosen if they had been fully informed.

Ethical issues

The primary goal of medicine is to benefit the patient, and if chemotherapy does not provide net benefit to the patient, it can ethically be withheld or withdrawn. The goal of care then shifts to palliation of symptoms by other means.[10]

Persisting with chemotherapy in patients who are dying promotes the myth that doctors can postpone death indefinitely. Doctors may continue to use such futile treatment for several reasons. They may fear litigation, they may have a sense of failing the patient, or they may simply lack the necessary communication skills.

The intention of the doctor in using palliative chemotherapy is ethically relevant to this debate. For the use of palliative chemotherapy to be justified, one or more of the following indications should apply:

- relief of symptoms
- prevention of problems
- prolongation of a good quality of life, not prolongation of suffering.

Psychosocial issues

Emotional strain can result from working closely with people who are suffering and facing a poor prognosis. Sometimes death follows soon after chemotherapy has been discontinued, and staff may be emotionally involved in the patient's struggle and death. It can be harder to cope with death when there was a chance of cure initially than if the condition was palliative from the time of diagnosis. A prolonged dying process may also be stressful for everyone concerned.

The transition to palliative care will change the patient's and family's view, and they may respond to this unpredictably. Patients need to understand their illness. In a study of lay 'common-sense' models of illness, Leventhal and colleagues found that most people who are trying to understand an illness seek information in the following areas.[11]

- *Identity*. What is it called? What are its symptoms?
- *Cause*. How did I come to have it?
- *Consequences*. How will it affect me? How will it affect those around me?
- *Timeline*. How will it change over time (e.g. resolving, chronic, remitting/ relapsing, deteriorating)?
- *Cure/control*. Can it be cured? If so, how? If not, can it be controlled? If so, how?

Despite the doctors' efforts to explain, patient misunderstandings can arise. Patients and their families may believe that the palliative chemotherapy may ultimately lead to cure, or cures may be sought when palliative care would be more appropriate. There may therefore be missed opportunities for the patient and their family to prepare for death. Research examining how people choose treatments shows that patients appear to be willing to undergo treatments for much less chance of benefit than most professionals would consider worthwhile.[12,13] A study by Slevin and colleagues showed that cancer patients have a different perspective to healthy people. The researchers asked the question 'What chance of controlling symptoms would encourage you to undergo palliative chemotherapy?'[13] The responses were as follows: healthy people, 50%; GPs, 25%; cancer doctors, 25%; cancer patients, 1%. It seems that there is a change in philosophy during illness. There may be a pressure on patients to provide some hope for themselves, and on the doctor to 'do something'.

Ajzen's theory of planned behaviour identifies the following as the main factors shaping attitude to an action, such as choosing to have a treatment.[14]

- What are the costs and benefits of this course of action?
- What do others (who matter to me) think about this?
- Will I be able to cope?

Decision making is not simply a question of informing the patient and leaving him to weigh up the costs and benefits. The patient is also influenced by the views of his friends and family. For example, he may feel under an obligation to accept chemotherapy to 'fight the cancer' for the sake of his family.

Maximising quality of life

Calman's model of quality of life describes a 'gap' between the reality of the patient's situation and their expectations, such that the greater the 'gap' the poorer their quality of life.[15] Therefore to maximise a patient's quality of life it is sometimes necessary to lower their expectations as well as ensuring that the patient's condition is as good as possible.

A sense of hope is one factor that gives life quality and makes it 'worth living'. Informing a patient that cure is no longer possible can be perceived as removing all hope. Feelings of hopelessness may lead to depression and the desire to die, so it is important that the patient has hopes for the future. There is a risk that unrealistic hopes may prevent the patient from dealing with their concerns, foster collusion and leave the patient feeling isolated. Realistic hopes may be hopes of pain relief or spending time at home, rather than of living for many years. The doctor's task is difficult – to foster the patient's hopes yet give the patient a chance to discuss their fears. In discussing hopes and fears, one strategy that the doctor and patient might employ is to 'hope for the best and prepare for the worst'. This strikes a balance between supporting the patient's hopes and allowing them to prepare for the end of their life if they wish to do so. It enables the doctor and patient to see that it is possible to be hopeful about many aspects of life, and at the same time to feel free to voice concerns about death.

Appropriate care

Involve specialist palliative care teams

Clear referral criteria for specialist palliative care should exist so that it can be introduced early enough in the illness trajectory. Raising awareness of the availability and role of palliative care during the curative phase may ease the transition into the palliative phase.

Specialist palliative care teams need to be part of routine care so that everyone (including the patient) is familiar with their role. Developing good working relationships over time with joint discussion of potential referrals between oncology and palliative care teams can help to deliver better continuity of care.

Addressing patients' fears

The patient's fears about palliative care need to be addressed. They require time to adjust to changes in the goals of care. Sheldon highlights the difficulties in making decisions because patients are inconsistent.[16] They may respond in one way during a discussion with an oncologist, but in a different way when discussing their treatment with a palliative care specialist. Different disciplines need to maintain clear channels of communication in order to acknowledge these difficulties and reach a consensus, rather than one discipline being perceived as critical of another.

A partnership between the patient and the doctor means that the two parties are working towards a common goal.[17] The relationship should be based on trust, and it should be acknowledged that patients are experts on many aspects of their lives.

Although the patient's needs are paramount, the views of relatives should also be taken into account. If there is a conflict between these views, time needs to be spent exploring the reasons for this and giving people time to adjust to new situations.

Communication issues

Medical language may reinforce remoteness, and financial restrictions and time constraints work against the humanisation of medical care – doctors and nurses are universally perceived to be busy. Another constraint on good communication is that doctors have their own fears of death, which may lead them to distance themselves from dying patients in order to retain control of their own feelings. Distancing may take the form of not making time available and of keeping the conversation limited to enquiries about symptoms and the treatment plan. There is also a risk that patient care of a non-technical nature may be delegated to the staff with least training.

In helping patients to understand their illness other team members should be involved in order to reinforce explanations. Access to written materials or the Internet may be helpful. Patients' understanding needs to be reviewed at each stage and the amount of information given matched to the individual's changing needs. The patient's assessments of their quality of life during and after palliative chemotherapy should be recorded in the clinical notes. The family's perceptions also need to be assessed, as their views may shape the patient's choice of treatment. Above all, professionals should be explicit about the realistic benefits and burdens of any proposed course of chemotherapy.

One way forward might be to give palliative chemotherapy a trial, and if there is no subsequent benefit then the focus of management should change to palliative care. Futile chemotherapy is easier to stop if the goals have been explained before treatment commences.

Patients may show resistance to accepting that the goal of care is palliative rather than curative. Sometimes the doctor feels more comfortable outlining available treatments than confronting difficult emotional issues surrounding death and dying. If chemotherapy fails to benefit the patient, the oncologist should express regret without giving an impression that they have failed. The patient should be reassured that although treatment of the cancer may have ceased, they will continue to receive support and palliative care.

Prognostic uncertainty

Prognostic uncertainty can be addressed by exploring the patient's concerns, acknowledging uncertainty and setting realistic goals. During the palliative phase of care, questions about the prognosis can be viewed as opportunities for the patient to discuss unfinished business and their fears about death.

Professionals need to improve their prognostic skills so that palliative care can be initiated at the most appropriate time.

Care for professionals

Healthcare professionals need to be aware of their boundaries, and should try to balance their work with the rest of their life. Reflective practice will encourage them to question themselves if they are thinking too much about a specific patient. If a doctor feels that he is getting too close to a particular patient, he should try to 'share the care' with other team members. Support for staff should be available in several forms, including formal supervision, appraisal, debriefing and taking time to discuss these issues in the team.

The patient's view

To 'suffer with' is the root meaning of the word 'compassion'. Suffering enforces isolation – severing people from family and social relationships. The presence of a doctor or nurse represents an opportunity to share one's vulnerability and suffering. Healthcare professionals need time to evaluate the patient's coping mechanisms. Time should be allowed to follow up and listen carefully to the patient's view. It is to be hoped that healthcare purchasers and providers will attach the same value to this quality time.

The patient must be able to feel in control. Treatment of the cancer may have ceased, but communication with the patient continues. Doctors need to be clear as to whose suffering it is that is being treated – the patient's, the family's or their own.

Conclusion

Many common solid tumours in adults are resistant to chemotherapy.[18] Using chemotherapy in a palliative manner to improve symptom control and maximise quality of life requires doctors to discuss the treatment options with their patients. Time should be allowed to ensure that patients fully understand these options. Decision making is complex, and individual patients' choices may differ from those of healthcare professionals. Patients and their families need time and privacy to assess the impact of the disease and potential treatments. Chemotherapy should not be given as a way of maintaining false hope, and doctors should stop treatments that are not of benefit to the patient. It is to be hoped that research will aid the selection of patients who are likely to benefit from palliative chemotherapy. At present the patients who are most likely to suffer toxicity effects are those with a poor performance status. Treatment regimes and investigations should be as simple as possible and should not impair the patient's quality of remaining life. The effect of the treatment on the patient's psychosocial well-being deserves as much attention as is given to their physical symptoms. Teamworking, and specifically the integration of oncology and specialist palliative treatments, should be valued in order to promote holistic patient care.

When a doctor's obligation to prolong life is balanced with his duty to relieve suffering, a peaceful death can be viewed as a success.

Key points

- The overall aim of chemotherapy for patients with advanced cancer should be to optimise the patients' quality of life.
- Clinicians may be caught in a dilemma between over-treating patients on the one hand and neglecting a remote chance of prolonged survival on the other.
- Doctors are neither legally nor morally obliged to offer futile treatments.
- Specialist palliative care teams need to be part of routine care so that everyone (including the patient) is familiar with their role.
- The involvement of patients is crucial both for reducing their sense of helplessness and for enhancing their feeling of control.

References

1 Rubens RD, Towlson KE, Ramirez AJ et al. (1992) Appropriate chemotherapy for palliating advanced cancer. *BMJ*. **304**: 35–40.
2 Ramirez AJ, Towlson KE, Leanin MS et al. (1998) Do patients with advanced breast cancer benefit from chemotherapy? *Lancet*. **347**: 724–8.
3 Jeffrey D (1995) Appropriate palliative care: when does it begin? *Eur J Cancer Care*. **4**: 122–6.
4 Gottlieb S (2001) Chemotherapy may be overused at the end of life. *BMJ*. **322**: 1267.
5 Colorectal Cancer Collaborative Group (2000) Palliative chemotherapy for advanced colorectal cancer: systematic review and meta-analysis. *BMJ*. **321**: 531–5.
6 Michael M and Zalcberg JR (2000) Chemotherapy for advanced colorectal cancer. *BMJ*. **321**: 521–2.

7 The A-M, Hak T, Koeter G *et al.* (2000) Collusion in doctor–patient communication about imminent death: an ethnographic study. *BMJ.* **321:** 1376–81.

8 Quirt CF, Mackillop WJ, Ginsburg AD *et al.* (1997) Do doctors know when their patients don't? A survey of doctor–patient communication in lung cancer. *Lung Cancer.* **18:** 1–20.

9 Silvestri G, Pritchard R and Welch HG (1998) Preferences for chemotherapy in patients with advanced non-small-cell lung cancer: descriptive study based on scripted interviews. *BMJ.* **317:** 771–5.

10 British Medical Association (2002) *Withholding and Withdrawing Life-Prolonging Medical Treatment. Guidance for decision making* (2e). British Medical Association, London.

11 Leventhal H, Meyer D and Nerenz D (1980) The common-sense representation of illness danger. In: S Rachman (ed.) *Contributions to Medical Psychology.* Jossey-Bass, San Francisco, CA.

12 Balmer CE, Thomas P and Osbourne RJ (2001) Who wants second-line chemotherapy? *Psycho-oncology.* **10:** 410–18.

13 Slevin ML, Stubbs L, Plant HJ *et al.* (1990) Attitudes to chemotherapy: comparing views of patients with cancer with those of doctors, nurses and the general public. *BMJ.* **300:** 1458–60.

14 Ajzen I (1985) From intention to action: a theory of planned behaviour. In: J Kuhl and J Beckman (eds) *Action Control: from cognition to behaviour.* Springer-Verlag, Berlin.

15 Calman KC (1984) Quality of life in cancer patients: a hypothesis. *J Med Ethics.* **10:** 124–7.

16 Sheldon F (1997) *Psychosocial Palliative Care.* Stanley Thornes Ltd, Cheltenham.

17 Coulter A (1999) Paternalism or partnership? *BMJ.* **319:** 719–20.

18 Kearsley JH (1994) Some basic guidelines on the use of chemotherapy for patients with incurable malignancy. *Palliat Med.* **8:** 11–17.

9 'Am I not worth treating?': Do Not Attempt Resuscitation decisions

We are born to do benefits.
Timon of Athens, I, ii.

Introduction

Essentially a doctor has the same responsibilities with regard to cardiopulmonary resuscitation (CPR) as they do in relation to any other treatment; namely to offer treatments that are likely to yield more benefit than harm. In the case of CPR the potential benefit is to prolong life. The possible harms include an undignified death, brain damage, or only a short survival without discharge from hospital.

CPR should only be provided when the benefits outweigh the harms. If it is judged to be futile then it should not be offered, as the doctor should always act in the patient's best interests. If there is any doubt about the balance between harm and benefit, the doctor must seek the patient's informed consent. A competent patient's informed refusal of CPR constitutes an advance directive and should be respected if the circumstances anticipated by the patient arise. A patient cannot compel the doctor to carry out CPR if the doctor's judgement is that the intervention is not in that patient's best interests. In dying patients in whom the harms caused by CPR may exceed the benefits, the doctor may discuss this with the patient before making a Do Not Attempt Resuscitation (DNAR) decision. However, in patients with advanced cancer, discussion of a DNAR decision is not always in a patient's best interests.

Legal issues concerning CPR

The Human Rights Act 1998 promotes a range of human rights which, in the context of CPR, aim to enhance human dignity and transparency in decision making. It is clear that in law no patient or carer can require a doctor to provide treatment that is contrary to his or her clinical judgement (i.e. contrary to the patient's best interests).[1] However, the law recognises that the assessment of best interests should include social welfare in its entirety.[2] If the patient is unable to make decisions, other interested parties should be consulted, except where that might harm the patient. In cases of dispute, consultation should take place with colleagues before deciding on best practice.

Guidelines on DNAR decisions are available from the British Medical Association, the Resuscitation Council (UK) and the Royal College of Nursing.[3] However, some of the most difficult dilemmas relate not to treatment specifically, but to communication issues with patients and their relatives.

Inappropriate CPR is common. It is undignified for patients and distressing for the hospital teams involved.[4] In the USA, hospital practice fully respects patient autonomy, and on every occasion the consent of the patient or surrogate consent is sought. Such an approach gives doctors no authority to refuse to give treatments that are in their judgments contraindicated.[5] This practice can be contrasted with that found in the UK, where policies vary depending on the patient's situation. For example, CPR is rarely performed in hospices or at home, whereas DNAR decisions are routinely considered in hospital wards, although they may not be discussed with the patient.[6] Thus doctors in the UK are enabled to reduce the inappropriate use of resuscitation, but at the expense of patient autonomy.

Guidelines

Policies on CPR and DNAR decisions need to be agreed locally in order to enhance clinical care. They should respect patient autonomy and protect individual doctors and nurses from criticism. The British Medical Association, Resuscitation Council and Royal College of Nursing guidelines are helpful in that they 'outline legal and ethical standards for planning patient care and decision making in relation to cardiopulmonary resuscitation'.[3] They aim to demystify the process by which decisions are made by emphasising the need to discuss the reasons for the DNAR order with the patient. However, there are a number of practical difficulties which are not addressed by these guidelines:

- the patient may demand CPR when the medical team considers that it would not be beneficial
- the role of the family
- notions of futility.

The guidelines do not clarify how the doctor should act if the patient demands that CPR be performed, when the doctor considers that it would be futile. Doctors have no legal obligation to offer any treatment which in their professional judgement they do not feel will benefit their patient.[7] However, the guidelines are ambiguous on this point, stating that:

> Doctors cannot be required to give treatment contrary to their clinical judgment but should, whenever possible, respect patients' wishes to receive treatment which carries only a very small chance of success or benefit.[3]

Discussion is necessary between doctors and those patients who request inappropriate treatment. Although refusing a treatment is emotionally difficult for doctors, particularly when it may appear that 'life is at stake', in patients with advanced cancer successful CPR cannot prolong life for more than a short time, nor can it improve its quality. Attempting CPR in such situations is medically inappropriate and promotes the myth that doctors can postpone death indefinitely.

Doctors may postpone discussion with the patient about a DNAR order until the patient is close to death, in order to avoid a refusal of the DNAR order. Delaying discussion in this way may mean that the patient is too frail to participate effectively in decision making.

If the patient is not competent to make decisions, the guidelines indicate that when a doctor is seeking information from the family, he should stress that they must consider what the patient's wishes would have been rather than what they would wish for the patient. Many relatives do not share this perception, and feel that they have a right to decide for their relative and even to demand CPR. This can leave them either in conflict with the medical staff or with feelings of guilt during their bereavement.[8]

Notions of the futility of CPR risk obscuring the decision-making process. Clearly, if the patient is dying from a terminal illness, CPR would be futile and inappropriate.[9] It is more helpful for the doctor to make a judgement about whether successful CPR is likely to benefit the patient.

Communication problems

Case history

Jill, a 55-year-old woman with advanced breast cancer, has been admitted for pain control. She has metastases in her lungs, liver and bones and is confined to bed most of the time. She has had surgery, radiotherapy, three different chemotherapy regimes and hormone therapy in the past. She is becoming weaker every day. Her doctor is asking her about her resuscitation status.

Dr Green: 'Good afternoon, Jill. I wonder if I could talk to you about your future care ... would that be OK?'

Jill: 'Yes, I would like to know what you are going to do to help me.'

Dr Green: 'The treatments which would help would be to get the balance of painkillers improved so that we could get you feeling much more comfortable.'

Jill: 'That would be great – are there any other things which might help?'

Dr Green: 'It would really help me if you could tell me what you think, Jill ... what do you hope for your future?'

Jill: 'I know there is no more chemo ... I would like to be able to spend some time at home with my family.'

Dr Green: 'I think that is a goal which we can work towards ... Another thing I would like your view on is that just as you realise that further chemo won't help you, there are other treatments which might do you more harm than good.'

Jill: 'What treatments?'

Dr Green: 'Well, the hospital has a policy that we need to discuss what you would want us to do in the unlikely event of you collapsing suddenly and your heart stopping ... would you wish to be resuscitated?'

Jill: 'Am I not worth treating?'

Dr Green: 'The situation is, Jill, that if resuscitating you had any real chance of success we would be advising you strongly to agree to it. However, in your situation the procedure has virtually no chance of success. I do want to emphasise that this decision would not alter the treatment to improve your pain control and to try to get you home.'

Jill: 'That was what I was really worried about. I don't want to be left on my own and no one bother.'

Dr Green: 'Of course not – we all want to help and focus on the things that we can do to improve your quality of life, but I did want to explain about the resuscitation. Have you any other questions about it?'

Jill: 'No, you've set my mind at rest. I was worried that if something happened I would be stuck on a ventilator with lots of tubes everywhere ... I would hate that.'

Talking about DNAR decisions with patients and relatives is not easy. Doctors may lack the language and skills necessary and may feel both a sense of failure and a fear of litigation. They may worry that the patient will be harmed by the discussion. Conversely, delaying the discussion until a time when the patient is frail often causes more distress. Another difficulty for doctors is that the discussion usually takes place when CPR is being withdrawn as a treatment option.[8]

The medical team should decide which member of the team should discuss these issues with the patient and relatives. The choice may not be the most senior physician but the team member with the most sensitive communication skills and the time available for discussion.

Patient recall of DNAR discussions may be poor, and doctors need to be aware of the need to give patients an opportunity to review their decision if they so wish.[10]

Improving the communication of DNAR decisions

The basic principles of good communication in difficult situations apply as much to DNAR decisions as to breaking bad news. The different stages of the process can be summarised as follows:

1 getting started
2 finding out how much the patient understands
3 finding out whether the patient wants this discussion
4 sharing the information
5 responding to the patient's feelings
6 planning and follow-up.

Clear and effective language

There is no one right way to initiate and conduct these discussions. However, the following suggestions may be helpful.[11]

Opening CPR discussions

- *'There are things that we can do to help you and things which are perhaps not so helpful.'* CPR is then discussed among other unhelpful options.
- *'We have a hospital policy that we discuss with everyone what they would want us to do in the unlikely event that they collapsed suddenly and their heart stopped. I am interested in your view.'*
- *'It would be good to hear from you what you think should happen in the future. Maybe a starting point is how you see things going from here.'*

Ending CPR discussions

Some phrases may allow the patient to stop the discussion if they wish:

- *'I realise that this is not an easy discussion.'*
- *'What is it about dying that you are frightened of?'*

The difference between a sudden collapse and the dying process needs to be made explicit.

One of the aims of the recent guidelines was to promote trust by demystifying the process of DNAR orders for patients. The British Medical Association guidance for decision making also recommends 'advanced planning for antici-pated medical events'.[3] If DNAR discussions took place within the context of general discussions about the aims of treatment at each hospital admission, some patients would have opportunities to discuss CPR at a time when it was considered an appropriate option.

As the disease progresses, the opportunity should be taken to discuss with patients the changing aims of treatment, quality-of-life issues and expectations of the future, in order to facilitate understanding and acceptance of a DNAR order when this becomes appropriate.

It is clear that many patients and relatives do not understand the nature of CPR and DNAR orders.[12] It is important to explain that this technique evolved in response to sudden cardiac arrest rather than as an intervention to be used in cases of advanced cancer. It should be emphasised that appropriate treatments continue after the DNAR order. This should be documented in the patient's notes alongside the DNAR order. Otherwise patients and their relatives may fear that a DNAR order will adversely affect the quality of their care.[13]

The critical issues in the communication of DNAR orders are the timing of the discussion and ensuring that the conversation relating to CPR forms part of a wider range of negotiations about the aims of care at the end of life.[8] In this way the patient will gain insight into and understanding of the fact that their disease is progressing. They will come to appreciate that the goals of care are now to provide comfort, to improve quality of life and to maintain dignity. Consequently, they will understand that invasive techniques such as surgery, powerful chemotherapy or CPR are no longer appropriate.

An interesting initiative is the development of a '*What Happens If ...*' leaflet that is given to patients on admission to hospital by the nursing staff. This leaflet is designed to raise the subject of CPR with patients and to legitimise discussion.[14]

Although relatives have no legal power to make decisions for another adult, staff should be available to discuss and explain the reasons why a DNAR decision would be appropriate in order to protect an individual from a futile and undignified treatment. They should also explain that all other treatments to ensure the comfort and dignity of the patient would be given.

Improving interprofessional communication

DNAR decisions should be recorded in the medical notes in a manner that reflects the professional's respect for the patient's dignity. It should be noted that there has been a clinical assessment by a senior clinician with responsibility for the patient's care, and that attempts at resuscitation would not benefit the patient. The DNAR order should be written legibly with no medical jargon, and should include the nature of the discussion with the patient and the family, the diagnosis, the time, the date of review, the date that the order was made and the signature of the responsible physician. If such discussion was either inappropriate or impossible, the reasons for this must be stated.

The decision must be shared between the medical and nursing teams. Procedures within teams for making decisions should be clear, and the views of the whole team need to be considered.

Just as the signed consent form is an acknowledgement that a process of informed consent has taken place, so too the documentation in the notes of a DNAR order is a record that the process of decision making has been carried forward in the appropriate way.

Improved communication may lead to many benefits.

- Fully informed consent may be achieved.
- Patients understand the severity of their condition and can plan accordingly at all stages of their illness.
- Patients are aware of which treatments are available.
- The family is informed and feels part of the decision-making process.
- There is an improved relationship with the patient.
- There is a clear idea of the goals of treatment.
- There is an awareness of full supportive measures.

Conclusion

In the last 30 years CPR has evolved. Initially it consisted of an intervention developed to treat the reversible precipitants of sudden death, indicated only in cases of acute insult to an otherwise healthy person, but now it has become a default measure that is employed in virtually all cases of death in hospital. Confusion exists in patients' minds between 'normal death' and cardiorespiratory arrest. Moreover, an increasing patient expectation of survival combined with fears about hospitals and a lack of trust in doctors has contributed to this excessive use of CPR. Society and doctors seem to have forgotten that death is an integral part of life. Smith acknowledges that 'doctors are often acutely aware of the limitations of what they can do, whereas patients – partly through the exaggeration of doctors – have inflated ideas of the power of medicine'.[15]

Most patients want their views taken into account when determining their treatment options, but feel that doctors should be the main decision makers. With regard to CPR, patients and relatives lack knowledge of the process involved. If they are to make autonomous judgements, patients need better education on CPR outcomes. This may be achieved by supplementing the discussion with written information. Each case should be considered carefully, and the same decision should never be applied to whole categories of patients. Respect for autonomy restricts CPR use when it is refused by the patient, but cannot create a 'right to CPR'.

A new way of approaching the issue of DNAR orders brings CPR into the everyday discussion with the patient while he or she is competent. As the disease progresses and the likely benefit of CPR becomes negligible, the ethical case for the doctor taking the responsibility for the decision becomes stronger (*see* Figure 9.1).[8]

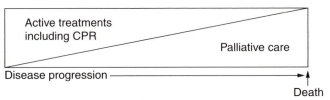

Figure 9.1 Disease progression and CPR

When considering ethical dilemmas, the model of the duties of autonomy, beneficence, non-maleficence and justice can be employed. In a clinical situation these duties often conflict, and Figure 9.2 illustrates a way in which the ethical duties may be prioritised in different clinical situations.

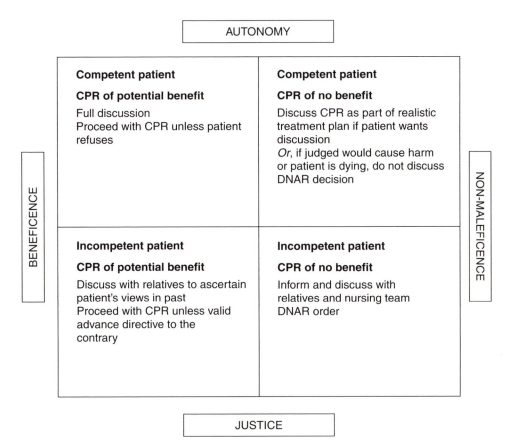

Figure 9.2 An ethical approach to DNAR decision making[8]

Such a model emphasises the necessity for adopting a case-by-case approach and for reviewing decision making frequently throughout the patient's illness. Patients and their relatives may feel that they are entitled to unlimited treatments.

It is necessary to examine whether it is ever unethical to discuss a DNAR decision with a competent patient. In general there is a strong ethical presumption in favour of discussing any proposed treatment with patients. However, a DNAR is a 'withholding of treatment' and therefore requires special attention. If a senior doctor feels that the patient may benefit from CPR, it is mandatory to discuss this with the patient. If he feels that, as a consequence of the severity of the patient's underlying clinical condition, CPR would have no benefit to them and harm resulting from such discussion would outweigh the benefits, there is no legal or moral imperative to discuss CPR with the patient.[8] Although early discussion with competent patients would form part of advance planning for end-of-life care, in a case of advanced terminal disease a DNAR decision may be made by the responsible consultant without the competent patient's involvement.[16]

Key points

- Talking to patients about DNAR decisions is difficult for many doctors.
- A doctor should not initiate any treatment, including CPR, if he or she does not believe that it will benefit the patient.
- Communication of DNAR decisions should occur as part of a wider discussion of treatment goals at an earlier stage in the patient's illness.
- An ethical framework may be of practical help in clarifying decision making.
- In a case of advanced terminal disease, a DNAR decision may be made by the responsible consultant without the competent patient's involvement.

References

1 *Re J (A minor) Wardship: Medical treatment* [1992] 4 All ER 614, CA.
2 *Re SL* [1999] 52 BMLR 124.
3 British Medical Association, Resuscitation Council and Royal College of Nursing (2001) *Decisions Relating to Cardiopulmonary Resuscitation: a joint statement.* British Medical Association, London.

4 De Vos R, de Haes HC, Koster RW *et al.* (1999) Quality of survival after cardiopulmonary resuscitation. *Arch Intern Med.* **159:** 249–54.

5 Mello M and Jenkinson C (1998) Comparison of medical and nursing attitudes to resuscitation and patient autonomy between a British and an American teaching hospital. *Soc Sci Med.* **46:** 415–24.

6 Willard C (2000) Cardiopulmonary resuscitation for palliative care patients: a discussion of ethical issues. *Palliat Med.* **14:** 308–12.

7 Luce JM (1995) Physicians do not have a responsibility to provide futile or unreasonable care if a patient or family insists. *Med Decision Making.* **21:** 141–9.

8 Reid C and Jeffrey D (2002) Do not attempt resuscitation decisions in a cancer centre: addressing difficult ethical and communication issues. *Br J Cancer.* **86:** 1057–60.

9 Ebell MH, Becker LA, Barry HC *et al.* (1998) Survival after in-hospital cardiopulmonary resuscitation: a meta-analysis. *J Gen Intern Med.* **13:** 805–16.

10 Stewart K and Spice C (2001) Not discussing decisions is often because of practicalities, not ageism (letter). *BMJ.* **322:** 104.

11 National Council for Hospice and Specialist Palliative Care Services (2003) *CPR: policies in action.* National Council for Hospice and Specialist Palliative Care Services, London.

12 Agard A, Hermeren G and Herlitz J (2000) Should cardiopulmonary resuscitation be performed on patients with heart failure? The role of the patient in the decision-making process. *J Intern Med.* **248:** 279–86.

13 Ebrahim S (2000) Do Not Resuscitate decisions: flogging dead horses or a dignified death? *BMJ.* **320:** 1155–6.

14 Attwood S, Anderson K and Mitchek T (2001) Discussing cardiopulmonary resuscitation with patients. *Br J Nurs.* **10:** 1201–7.

15 Smith R (2000) A good death. *BMJ.* **320:** 129–30.

16 Dunphy K (2000) Futilitarianism: knowing how much is enough in end-of-life care. *Palliat Med.* **14:** 313–22.

10 'Water, water everywhere': Artificial nutrition and hydration at the end of life

Men so noble,
However faulty, yet should find respect
For what they have been: 'tis a cruelty
To load a falling man.

King Henry VIII, V, iii.

Background

The question of whether dying patients should be given fluids by artificial means has generated a debate that has ethical, legal, physiological and emotional dimensions.

The primary goal of terminal care is the patient's dignity and comfort. For some patients, not taking food or drink may be part of the natural dying process. However, there is a strong feeling that dying patients should be offered food and water. Furthermore, there is concern that a patient whose wishes cannot be determined may be suffering because they are hungry or thirsty. However, in some situations, providing artificial nutrition and hydration can cause further suffering.

Doctors must act for the benefit of the patient and with the patient's consent.[1] Benefit in this context refers not to prolongation of life but to relief of suffering. The General Medical Council (GMC) guidelines recognise that a treatment may not be worth having if it confers no benefit on the patient, if it only prolongs the dying process and causes unnecessary distress to the patient.[2] In situations where the patient is unable to give or withhold consent, the doctor must act in what is judged to be the patient's best interests.

When considering artificial hydration the situation is more complex, as some believe that the provision of water is 'basic care' which healthcare professionals have a duty to provide, rather than a 'treatment' which may or may not confer a benefit on the patient. This differentiation is arbitrary, since it is possible for a patient to refuse to have an intervention described as 'basic care'.

Competent patients

The courts have granted competent adult patients an absolute right to refuse treatment even if non-treatment means that death will occur.[3] This view takes into account the patient's experience of their illness and treatment.

Legally, patients have a right to refuse medical interventions which would have the effect of shortening their life, but there is no right to demand life-shortening interventions.[4] As the case of Diane Pretty confirmed, a patient has no 'right' to assisted suicide.[5] There is no legal 'right to die'.

Incompetent patients

Advance directives

If a patient is not competent and has made an advance directive to refuse treatment when previously competent, that directive is legally binding, provided that the advance refusal is clearly established and applicable to the circumstances that have occurred and that there is no reason to believe that the patient has changed their mind.[2,6] However, an inevitable consequence of accepting an advance directive is the doctor's uncertainty as to whether the patient might have changed their view later.

Although a competent patient has a right to refuse a treatment, the same cannot be said for a demand for a particular treatment. The GMC guidance also states that 'where a patient wishes to have a treatment that – in the doctor's considered view – is not clinically indicated, there is no ethical or legal obligation on the doctor to provide it'.[2] An interesting development in recent case law is that a patient can make an advance directive that artificial hydration be provided even if the doctors feel that it would not be in the patient's best interests.[7] A high court ruling concluded that in the case of Burke the current GMC guidance is unlawful. Mr Justice Munby ruled that the patient could insist on receiving artificial nutrition and hydration, and in the subsequent event of the patient becoming incompetent to make decisions, doctors would be bound by law to give the nutrition and hydration. Although patients have always had the right to refuse treatment and to make an advance directive to that effect, they have never before had a right to insist that a doctor provide a treatment that they consider not to be in the patient's best interests.[7]

The GMC have appealed against this judgement, since establishing a right to require treatment could result in doctors being legally bound to provide treatments which they consider to be contrary to the patient's best interests.[8]

When no advance directive exists

If no advance directive exists, the doctor must act in the patient's best interests. It is not in the patient's best interests to be subjected to treatment that is futile or that would inflict excessive burdens on the patient.

Role of the relatives

Relatives cannot give or withhold consent on behalf of another adult, but they may provide information to help the doctor to decide whether the patient would have considered artificial hydration to be beneficial. If a patient lacks the capacity to decide, the doctor, the healthcare team and the patient's family should try to reach a consensus about treatment.[2] In the unlikely event of it being difficult to reach agreement, legal advice should be sought.

A relative may insist that the patient is given fluids. However, they may change their request if they are given time and support to understand that intravenous fluids will not have an effect on thirst, but that good mouth care can alleviate this symptom. Offers of oral hydration and nutrition must continue.

It is important that relatives understand that when the patient is unable to communicate, their contribution to decision making is to enlighten the medical staff as to what the patient would have wanted if they were competent. What a relative might wish for him- or herself is not the issue.

Best interests

Before deciding in an individual case whether to initiate artificial hydration in the terminal stages of illness, the doctor needs to assess the burdens and possible benefits of the intervention.

Potential benefits of artificial hydration

These include the following:

- prolonging life
- correcting dehydration
- relieving thirst
- restoring consciousness
- doing something – not abandoning the patient
- correcting blood biochemistry.

The correction of electrolyte imbalance in terminally ill patients is rarely of benefit, since both patients who are artificially hydrated and those who are not often have only moderately disturbed electrolyte balances. Some degree of dehydration is a normal part of the dying process, and this is more effectively managed by meticulous attention to the patient's mouth care. Giving artificial hydration may confer a psychological benefit, reassuring doctors and relatives that 'something is being done'.

Potential burdens of artificial hydration

These include the following:

- prolonging the dying process
- causing discomfort
- necessitating hospital admission
- creating a barrier between the patient and their relatives
- sending a confusing message – medical interventions are continuing yet the patient is dying.

Healthcare professionals need to ask themselves whether artificial hydration given to correct electrolyte disturbance is going to maintain the comfort of the patient. Fears of being perceived to be abandoning the patient or neglecting a duty of care may prompt doctors to prescribe artificial hydration. Fluids when prescribed are often given in amounts that do not correct dehydration and which certainly have no nutritional benefit, although relatives often talk of 'drip feeding'.

If a patient complains of thirst, this is best managed by mouth care rather than by administering intravenous fluids.

Disease trajectories

In a study of the withholding of artificial hydration from elderly patients with dementia, two illness trajectories were identified,[9] namely a slow downward curve and interruption.

Slow downward curve

The gradual deterioration was regarded as part of the natural course of the disease. Care depended on nursing staff, and artificial nutrition and hydration were hardly ever used.

Interruption

Acute illnesses such as infection often interrupted the gradual deterioration. These were considered to be reversible and medically treatable. In these cases artificial nutrition and hydration were given. At a later stage, if the patient was dying, the illness process was then considered to be irreversible, and artificial nutrition and hydration were not given.

Benefit to the patient

Parenteral nutrition may prolong survival in a patient with advanced cancer, but it can also cause further suffering and make hospitalisation necessary. It is rarely used in this situation. Rehydration may be of benefit if the underlying condition is reversible. However, in many cases it too can add to the patient's distress.

It may be emotionally more difficult for healthcare professionals to withdraw hydration from a patient than to decide not to provide it in the first place. This should not be used as a reason for failing to initiate a treatment which could be of some benefit to a patient.[2]

A trial of treatment

In cases where the value of artificial nutrition and hydration is unclear it may be possible to initiate a time-limited trial of hydration and/or feeding to assess whether it confers any benefit.

Prognosis

Decisions relating to artificial feeding and hydration in patients with advanced cancer must not only be based on the doctor's estimate of the prognosis but also take into account the patient's views and those of their relatives. Although guidelines are welcome, they cannot replace a careful assessment of the individual patient.

Communication

The key to improving practice is effective communication both among members of the healthcare team and between the team and the patient and relatives. In the majority of cases patients will make their own choices, but in situations where they are unable or choose or do not wish to decide for themselves, the doctor should be able to make a decision which both the relatives and other healthcare professionals feel comfortable with because they all believe it to be in the best interests of the patient.[10]

Case history

Bill is a 60-year-old man with oesophageal cancer and widespread metastases in his liver and lungs. He has been admitted to hospital and is now weak, confined to bed and cannot swallow more than occasional sips of water. He is receiving analgesics and anti-emetics through a syringe driver. His condition is deteriorating every day. He is confused and sleepy and is unable to take part in any conversation.

His wife Betty cannot accept that he is dying, and insists that he should receive intravenous fluids.

Dr White: 'Thank you for coming to speak to me about Bill. Can you tell me a bit more about your concerns?'

Betty: 'He is starving to death. I can't understand why he has not got a drip feed.'

Dr White: 'I would like to explain a bit more, but before I do are there any other concerns?'

Betty: 'Well, he is so weak, it's the lack of food ... he is not getting stronger ... how can he manage without food?'

Dr White: 'You are right, he is getting weaker. Before I explain about the feeding, could you tell me what you understand about Bill's illness?'

Betty: 'I know that the cancer has spread and that it is not going to go away, but I don't understand why you are not feeding him so that he can get stronger and fight the cancer ... he must be very thirsty and all he's getting are sips of water.'

Dr White: 'Let me explain. Bill is not thirsty. The nurses, like you, take particular care to make sure that his mouth is moist and clean and that he is still taking sips. All his care is directed towards making him as comfortable as possible since he is much weaker now because his cancer is more advanced.'

Betty: 'I just want him to be comfortable ... I know he is much weaker ...' (*cries*)

Dr White: (*allows silence*) 'It must be very difficult for you to see Bill like this.'

Betty: 'We had so many plans ... after the treatment ... we were going to visit our son in Australia ... it's not fair ...'

Dr White: 'I agree, it's very hard ... but we both can see that Bill is dying and we want him to be as comfortable and dignified as possible. Giving him a drip would not make him feel any more comfortable, and might make him feel worse. Some dehydration is a natural part of dying.'

Betty: 'I can see what you are saying makes sense. Bill would never have wanted to go on like this ...'

Dr White: 'I am grateful to you for voicing your concerns. As Bill gets weaker I need you to tell me whether we are caring for him in the way both he and you would wish. Since Bill cannot tell us what he wants because he is so weak, I need to be guided by you, although the responsibility for the treatment decisions is mine.'

Betty: 'Thank you for taking the time to explain. I am relieved that we are not neglecting him.'

Dr White: 'This is a situation which we review each day. If a time comes when it looks as though there could be any benefit to Bill from giving intravenous fluids I would be happy to discuss this with you. Sometimes if there is any doubt a short trial of fluids can be given to see if there is any improvement in the patient's symptoms. These fluids can then be stopped if there is no benefit. However, I feel that in Bill's case he is dying – it is highly unlikely that his condition will improve or necessitate intravenous fluids.'

Betty: 'I am much happier now that I have had a chance to talk ... thank you for listening. I just find it so difficult to accept that he is dying.'

Doctors need to discover what the patient wants. If the patient is not competent and no advance directive exists, the relatives may have relevant information regarding the patient's wishes. The healthcare professionals need to provide clear information about the advantages and disadvantages of artificial hydration. The feelings and concerns of the relatives require careful exploration. Doctors need to be perceived as listening to the relatives' views and being prepared to change their minds.

Everyone concerned needs to be aware of the need for continuing palliative care and that withdrawing hydration should not be perceived as abandoning the patient. The family needs to be clear about the goals of care and what support they can receive. As in any decision about treatment, regular review of the patent's condition is essential in order to determine whether the goals of treatment have altered and whether the present management plan remains appropriate.

Key points

- The primary goal of terminal care is the patient's dignity and comfort.
- Doctors must act for the benefit of the patient and with the patient's consent.
- A treatment may not be worth having if it confers no benefit on the patient, if it only prolongs the dying process and if it causes unnecessary distress to the patient.
- A competent patient has an absolute right to refuse to consent to treatment for any reason, even when that decision may lead to his or her own death.
- Some degree of dehydration is a normal part of the dying process.
- In cases where the value of artificial nutrition and hydration is unclear, it may be possible to initiate a time-limited trial of hydration.

References

1 British Medical Association (2002) *Withholding and Withdrawing Life-Prolonging Medical Treatment. Guidance for decision making* (2e). British Medical Association, London.
2 General Medical Council (2002) *Withholding and Withdrawing Life-Prolonging Treatments: good practice in decision making.* General Medical Council, London.
3 *Re B* [2002] 2 All ER 449.

4 Keown J (2003) Medical murder by omission? The law and ethics of withholding and withdrawing treatment and tube feeding. *Clin Med JRCPL*. **3**: 460–3.

5 *Pretty v United Kingdom* [2002] 35 EHRR1.

6 *Re T* [1992] 3 WLR 782.

7 *R (Burke) v GMC* [2004].

8 Gillon R (2004) Why the GMC is right to appeal over life-prolonging treatment. *BMJ*. **329**: 810–11.

9 The A-M, Pasman R, Onwuteaka-Phillipsen BD *et al*. (2002) Withholding the artificial administration of fluids and food from elderly patients with dementia: ethnographic study. *BMJ*. **325**: 1326–9.

10 Farsides B (1999) Withholding or withdrawing treatment. *Int J Palliat Nurs*. **5**: 296–7.

11 'Help me to die': Euthanasia

> I cannot tell what you and other men
> Think of this life.
>
> *Julius Caesar*, I, ii.

Background

A doctor who intentionally kills a patient by the administration of drugs at the patient's voluntary and competent request is performing *euthanasia*. If the doctor helps a patient to commit suicide by providing drugs for self-administration, at that person's voluntary and competent request, then he or she is participating in *physician-assisted suicide*.[1]

The morality of euthanasia has been debated for years, but in recent times issues of patient choice, autonomy and the increasing ability of medical technology to prolong not only survival but also the process of dying have combined to bring this debate to public attention. A House of Lords Select Committee has produced a report on the Assisted Dying for the Terminally Ill Bill.[2] Although the members of the committee were divided, the report recommends that euthanasia and physician-assisted suicide be considered separately, and that the report be considered as a basis for debate if the issue is raised in Parliament in the future.

Both euthanasia and physician-assisted suicide have been legal in Belgium and the Netherlands since 2002. Physician-assisted suicide, but not euthanasia, was legalised in Oregon in 1997. Furthermore, Article 115 of the Swiss penal code condones assisting suicide for altruistic reasons. It does not require the involvement of a physician, nor that the patient be terminally ill.

The argument concerning the legalisation of euthanasia and physician-assisted suicide has polarised into two opposing views – 'for' and 'against'. The principal arguments for euthanasia and physician-assisted suicide concern respect for autonomy and the relief of pain and suffering. The arguments against them concern the intrinsic wrongness of killing, the integrity of the medical profession and the potential for abuse (the 'slippery-slope' argument).[3]

There is a clear distinction between euthanasia and the withholding or withdrawal of life-prolonging treatment. The withdrawal of life-prolonging treatments when these are not of benefit to the patient recognises the limits of a doctor's power and allows the patient to die as a consequence of their underlying disease. This is clinically, ethically and legally different from deliberate ending of life as in euthanasia.[4]

Developing the arguments surrounding legislation

The appropriate scope of respect for autonomy

The appropriate scope of respect for autonomy requires further scrutiny in relation to the wider interests of vulnerable patients and society.[3,5] In a society that legalises euthanasia on the basis of compassion, it is naive to imagine that the barrier to non-voluntary euthanasia would remain. If compassion is to be shown to patients who are able to request euthanasia, by the same argument it should be extended to those who are dying from physical and mental handicaps who are unable to request euthanasia.[4]

Thus there is a danger of reclassifying death from euthanasia and physician-assisted suicide as a potential moral good.[5] In the Netherlands, death and 'medicalised killing' are considered to be in the best interests not only of competent patients who request them, but also of incompetent patients, if the doctor(s) judge those patients to be suffering or in possession of a life that is no longer worth living.[6] However, medicalised killing is not the best treatment for suffering, particularly when poor clinical care has reduced a patient's dignity or if social isolation has led to a loss of personal relationships.

Clinical experience shows that if there is proper provision of palliative care services, and adequate and timely access to practical and necessary support for patients and their relatives, persistent requests for euthanasia are infrequent. Where such requests do exist, the solution lies in providing support and the best possible care to engage with issues such as hopelessness and suffering, not in euthanasia or physician-assisted suicide.

Relief of suffering

Relief of suffering is an important goal of medical care. However, palliative care cannot and does not claim to be able to relieve all suffering. There is no type of care that could ever alleviate all suffering (especially some expressions of social, psychological and spiritual distress). The first step in addressing suffering is to ensure that effective support and skilled interventions are available. If euthanasia was to be legalised, there is a risk that suffering in vulnerable patients and their families could be increased by reducing trust, increasing fear and inhibiting patients from disclosing their concerns to doctors and other healthcare professionals.

It is impossible to objectively determine the severity of suffering. Suffering is a subjective concept that is determined by a host of factors, including the patient, society, healthcare professionals and the level of support available.

Caring for dying patients can provoke feelings of hopelessness and failure among doctors.[7] In some cases the patient's request for euthanasia may be an indication that others have despaired of the patient.[4] It would be unwise to give doctors legal power to perform euthanasia when some physicians are insensitive to the psychological complexities of communicating with dying patients.[8]

Patients' views

There is a lack of reliable evidence as to how most dying patients feel about euthanasia and physician-assisted suicide. The evidence that does exist indicates that requests for euthanasia and physician-assisted suicide relate to feelings of 'disintegration', resulting from loss of function and from a 'loss of community' (the loss of close personal relationships). These factors combine to create a feeling of 'loss of self'.[9] The decision to proceed with euthanasia or physician-assisted suicide could thus change with alterations in an individual's social circumstances, independently of disease progression.[9]

Existing studies of patients' reasons for requesting euthanasia or physician-assisted suicide suffer from significant methodological weaknesses. They describe features such as depression, hopelessness, psychological distress and need for social support. However, the precise way in which these factors lead people to request euthanasia or physician-assisted suicide has not been explained.[10] What does seem to be clear is that the relevant factors can change as the patient approaches death.[11]

Legislation abroad

Looking at the effect of different laws in different countries will not necessarily predict the effect of legalising euthanasia in the UK. However, the Dutch data from 2001 give cause for concern.[6,12] Euthanasia was performed in 2.6% of all deaths, physician-assisted suicide in 0.2% of all deaths and 'life-terminating treatment, *where there is no explicit request*' in 0.7% of all deaths (almost 1000 patients per year).

Legislation has not been able to prevent life-terminating treatment without consent in the Netherlands. Furthermore, there is evidence that approximately 50% of cases of euthanasia are not reported by doctors, who feel that it is a private matter between themselves and the patient.[1,13] Thus the exact extent of euthanasia being performed without consent is unknown.

Implications for medical practice

The potential effect of legalising euthanasia on relationships between patients and their doctors should also be considered. The risk of losing trust and damaging care is high. Euthanasia and physician-assisted suicide would become legitimate treatment options that doctors would be obliged to raise with all dying patients. It is difficult to envisage how any proposed law would be enacted if the majority of doctors conscientiously object to performing euthanasia and physician-assisted suicide. The proposed legislation provided no details about the way in which euthanasia or physician-assisted suicide was to be performed. Problems may occur, and the Dutch experience shows that complications such as failure of completion, myoclonus and vomiting may occur in both physician-assisted suicide and euthanasia in 3–16% of patients, causing distress for patients.[14]

Clinical experience indicates that consultants are often inaccurate in their estimation of a patient's prognosis. Defining the terminal phase is often much more difficult than people might imagine, particularly in patients with non-malignant disease such as cardiac or respiratory failure.[15]

Commonly in clinical practice many patients are apprehensive and may be reluctant to accept palliative care. However, they almost always change their minds once they *experience* this type of care. Thus it may be that many patients who request euthanasia might initially reject palliative care when given basic information about it at a single interview.

Thou shalt not kill

There are strong cultural, moral and legal prohibitions on killing. Legislation might change the way in which society views sick and dying people. They may come to be regarded as an inconvenience and euthanasia as a solution to the challenges and costs of caring for the vulnerable. Patients may feel more of a burden to their families and society, and therefore may feel that they ought to request euthanasia. Legislation could actually increase the mental suffering of patients who would not necessarily want euthanasia, but who need care and can easily be distressed by feeling a burden. Roy questions whether society's resistance to non-voluntary euthanasia would soften as people became more accustomed to various modifications and extensions of voluntary euthanasia.[4] For all of these reasons it is vital to maintain a prohibition on the legalisation of euthanasia.

Responding to a request for euthanasia

Individual requests for euthanasia and physician-assisted suicide are complex in origin and demand careful attention with open and sensitive communication. The complexity of the notion of a 'loss of self' means that there is a need for clinicians to consider the evaluation of a request for euthanasia or physician-assisted suicide as an important clinical skill.[16] Sensitive exploration of the request can help to identify the real needs of the individual patient. The request for euthanasia or physician-assisted suicide seems to point to a series of concerns that the patient has about dying, relating to loss of self, loss of dignity and the social context of dying. Understanding these concerns may help to improve the care of dying patients. Performing euthanasia or physician-assisted suicide is no part of the duty of a doctor specialising in palliative medicine. It is imperative that patients, their families and the public are clear that palliative care is completely different to and separate from euthanasia and physician-assisted suicide.

In responding to the patient's request, the initial assessment interview is important in enabling a discussion of relevant care. However, assessment in specialist palliative care depends upon continuity of care and is an ongoing dynamic activity. It is unrealistic to imagine that a single consultation with a patient could reveal all of the factors underlying a request for euthanasia or physician-assisted suicide. It may take days or even weeks to establish a sufficiently trusting relationship with some patients. Compounding these difficulties is the lack of time and continuity, and the fact that many patients have a number of attending physicians and other healthcare professionals who are necessarily involved in their care.

The assessment of the euthanasia request can create a barrier that subtly alters the doctor–patient relationship and may paradoxically hamper the possibility of discussing the hopes and fears that gave rise to the euthanasia request. Sometimes it can be even more difficult to assess a patient's needs when the goal of euthanasia dominates discussion.

Communication and the euthanasia request

Case history

Jill, a 32-year-old teacher, is married with two daughters, Anna (aged 10 years) and Sophie (aged 5 years). She has advanced breast cancer with widespread metastases, and she has been admitted to hospital for a trial of third-line chemotherapy. She is in a single room adjacent to the ward and has become increasingly withdrawn. She has refused any food or drink and has asked if her drip could be taken down. Dr Smith, the oncologist, asks her what she would like to do.

Jill: 'Help me to die.'
Dr Smith: 'Jill, I can see that you are distressed about the difficult situation that you are facing. Of course we can take down the IV fluids if you wish, but do you want to talk a bit more about how you are feeling?'
Jill: (*silence ... long pause*).
Dr Smith: 'Look, we really want to help. I have colleagues who work in a palliative care team who could help you. Would you agree to see one of the team?'
Jill: (*silence ... long pause ... nods*).
Dr Smith: 'Thank you – I will ask Dr Green to see you this evening.'

Referral

Referral to a specialist palliative care team may be a problem. In the case described above, Jill has never met anyone from the specialist palliative care team before. Earlier referral to specialist teams allows the development of trusting relationships when there is no 'crisis', and facilitates later communication when difficult issues arise.

Case history

Dr Green walks along the corridor towards Jill's room, passing an elderly couple and two young girls. He knocks and enters Jill's room.

Dr Green: 'Good evening, Mrs Wood. My name is Dr Green – I am part of the palliative care team. Dr Smith asked me to see you. Is this OK?'

Jill: 'Yes ... please call me Jill.'

Dr Green (*sitting down alongside Jill's bed*):   'Dr Smith told me about your medical treatment, and I would like to hear from you how you feel things are going.'

Jill: 'I just want you to help me to die.'

Dr Green: (*silence ... pause*) 'Jill, I can see how difficult this must be for you ... could you please tell me a little more about what you want us to do?'

Jill: 'There's no point ... I just want it all to stop ... the chemo ... the drips ... everything. Please ... won't you help me to die?'

Dr Green: 'You know that doctors can't deliberately end your life, but could we look at some things that we can do to make things a bit easier for you?'

Jill: (*silence ... long pause*) 'I miss Anna and Sophie so much ... but they mustn't see me like this' (*pause*). 'I wish I was at home, but my parents can't cope with me and the girls ... are you sure you can't give me an injection?'

Dr Green: 'No, I can't do that, but I think we can work out some things that will help you to feel less awful. I think I saw your parents waiting outside the day room. Would it be all right for me to invite them to join us, to see how we can help to address some of your concerns?'

Jill: 'I don't want to bother them. Dad has a weak heart ...'

Dr Green: 'OK, I understand what you are saying ... but I think they would want to help.'

Jill: 'All right, but I can't face the children like this.'

Dr Green: 'That's OK, we can take one step at a time. Thank you for talking to me, I will make sure that the drip is taken down, and I know that there is no more chemo planned. Let's spend some time now looking at how we can achieve some of the things you want.'

Jill: 'Thank you ... please leave the door open ...'

Dr Green: (*leaving*) 'I will be back in a few minutes with your parents.'

The above case history illustrates the use of silence to allow reflection, to acknowledge the severity of the situation and to develop empathy. The doctor takes time to introduce himself and to request the *patient's* permission to have the interview. This is a small but significant sign of respect for autonomy, and shows the patient that the doctor wishes her to have as much control as possible. The request for euthanasia can be seen as a symptom that demands exploration in a sensitive way. Clarification of ambiguities such as 'help … to die', exploration of the reasons for the request and a genuine attempt to understand some of the distress the patient is experiencing are integral to the assessment interview. There can be no fixed rules on how to respond to a patient in such distress other than to follow the patient's agenda. This kind of communication requires the doctor to be sensitive to any cues that the patient offers. Cues may signal unrelieved pain, depression, distress, fear of loss of control and social concerns. In the above case history, Jill is voicing her real concerns, which centre around her children, her parents and her place of care.

Case history

Dr Green talks to Jill's parents, who want to help to look after her and understand that she is dying. They say that the children are missing their mother but have been told that they can't visit her because 'Mummy is too poorly'. Her parents return with Dr Green to see Jill. As they enter the room her father comments 'You look better for having the door open, Jill!' and goes on to explain to Dr Green that Jill has always had a fear of enclosed rooms since she became trapped in a lift as a child. The doctor, Jill and her parents talk about Jill's future care and the range of support that can be offered at home. Jill becomes aware that there is nursing and social support available which would enable her to enjoy some time with her family in her own home.

The next day Dr Green looks into a four-bedded ward to which Jill has been moved. Anna is showing her mother her school photo and Sophie is sitting on the bed drinking a can of Coke.

Dr Green: 'I'm sorry to interrupt but I wanted to say goodbye … I have not met your girls – hello, Anna … hello, Sophie. It's great to hear that Mummy is coming home tomorrow.'

Jill: 'Yes, I met the district nurse this morning – she came here to the ward to see me … and a Macmillan nurse is coming in on Monday.'

> Dr Green: 'I will keep in touch with your GP, Dr Symes, who I know is popping in as soon as you get home. If you need any help she is your first point of call, and she wants to know if any problems should crop up.'

The discussion with Jill's parents allowed the doctor to gain a greater understanding of the unique combination of factors contributing to Jill's distress. The simple acts of opening the door to her room, facilitating her transfer back into a ward and encouraging her to see her children gave Jill a sense of being valued, involved in the life of others and having her fears addressed. She felt in control yet she also felt supported to be able to return home with her family.

The request for euthanasia may be regarded as a cry for help. The precipitating factors change during the course of the illness, but they demand the skilled attention of healthcare professionals.

Conclusions

Palliative care is concerned with enabling patients with advanced life-threatening conditions to have the best possible quality of life until they die. Clinical experience and research suggest that the majority of requests for euthanasia or physician-assisted suicide arise as a result of poor symptom control, depression, poor social and family support and a loss of autonomy. Palliative care concentrates on improving these aspects of the patient's life, and the provision of such care should be the starting point for any debate on euthanasia, physician-assisted suicide and 'assisted dying'.

Palliative care involves working closely with patients and their families' suffering. When a patient is in the terminal phase of illness then the goal of care is to enhance the dignity of the individual.

The interests of dying patients, their families and wider society would be best served by increasing access to palliative care, improving communication between healthcare professionals and patients, gaining a better understanding of the needs of dying patients and informing the public about these highly complex issues in an honest way.

Key points

- Euthanasia and physician-assisted suicide should not be legalised.
- It is important to make a clear distinction between euthanasia and the withholding or withdrawal of life-prolonging treatment.
- There is a danger of reclassifying death from euthanasia and physician-assisted suicide as a potential moral good.
- The first step in addressing suffering is to ensure that effective support and skilled interventions are available to those who require them, rather than introducing a way to end these individuals' lives.
- There is little reliable evidence as to how most dying patients feel about euthanasia and physician-assisted suicide.
- The decision to proceed with euthanasia could change as a result of meaningful alterations in an individual's social circumstances independently of disease progression.
- Clinicians should consider the evaluation of a request for euthanasia or physician-assisted suicide as an important clinical skill.
- It is imperative that patients, their families and the public are clear that palliative care is completely different and separate from euthanasia and physician-assisted suicide.

References

1 Matersteedt LJ (2003) Palliative care on the 'slippery slope' towards euthanasia. *Palliat Med*. 17: 387–92.
2 House of Lords Select Committee Report (2005) *Assisted Dying for the Terminally Ill Bill*. The Stationery Office, London.
3 Battin MP (2003) Euthanasia and physician-assisted suicide. In: HO La Folette (ed.) *The Oxford Handbook of Practical Ethics*. Oxford University Press, Oxford.
4 Roy DJ (2004) Euthanasia. In: D Doyle *et al.* (eds) *Oxford Textbook of Palliative Medicine* (3e). Oxford University Press, Oxford.
5 George R (2004) *Case against the Assisted Dying Bill* (personal communication).
6 Keown J (2002) The Dutch in denial? In: *Euthanasia, Ethics and Public Policy*. Cambridge University Press, Cambridge.
7 Cherny NI, Coyle C and Foley KM (1994) Suffering in the advanced cancer patient: a definition and taxonomy. *J Palliat Care*. 10: 57–70.
8 Ramirez AJ (1996) Mental health of hospital consultants: the effects of stress and satisfaction at work. *Br J Cancer*. 78: 1488–94.

9 Lavery JV *et al.* (2001) Origins of the desire for euthanasia and assisted suicide in people with HIV-1 or AIDs: a qualitative study. *Lancet.* **358:** 362–7.

10 Mak YY *et al.* (2003) Patients' voices are needed in debates on euthanasia. *BMJ.* **327:** 213–15.

11 Chochinov HM *et al.* (1999) Will to live in the terminally ill. *Lancet.* **354:** 816–19.

12 Onwuteaka-Phillipsen BD *et al.* (2003) Euthanasia and other end-of-life decisions in the Netherlands in 1990, 1995 and 2001. *Lancet.* **362:** 395–9.

13 Haverkate I *et al.* (2000) Refused and granted requests for euthanasia and assisted suicide in the Netherlands: interview study with structured questionnaire. *BMJ.* **321:** 865.

14 Groenewood JH *et al.* (2000) Clinical problems with the performance of euthanasia and physician-assisted suicide in the Netherlands. *NEJM.* **342:** 551–6.

15 Glare P *et al.* (2004) Predicting survival in patients with advanced disease. In: D Doyle *et al.* (eds) *Oxford Textbook of Palliative Medicine* (3e). Oxford University Press, Oxford.

16 Back AL *et al.* (2001) Desire for physician-assisted suicide: requests for a better death? *Lancet.* **358:** 368.

Part 3

Good practice

12 The patient's choice

Sorrow concealed, like an oven stopp'd,
Doth burn the heart to cinders where it is.
Titus Andronicus, II, iv.

Introduction

The central theme in this book has been consideration of the individual patient when discussing both ethical dilemmas and difficult communication issues. Patient-centred care involves not only an understanding of the patient's clinical requirements, but also an exploration of their attitudes, beliefs and fears. The doctor comes to know the patient as a fellow human being.[1] This chapter focuses on ethics and communication from the patient's perspective. Assumptions that the healthcare professional is best placed to make decisions on the patient's behalf, without his or her involvement, are questioned. The tendency now is for appropriate models of decision making to be based on a partnership between the patient and the healthcare professionals.

Communication

A study of palliative care patients found that these patients received information from two main sources.[2] First, they were given information by healthcare professionals at the time of their initial diagnosis, or when there was a change in their condition or some new information emerged. Secondly, they received information from friends, family and the media.

Many patients were dissatisfied with the process of communication. They needed time to assimilate new information. If trust was lost during the initial consultation, this remained an issue for patients at later stages of their illness. There is an important lesson here for medical practice. The initial consultation during which the bad news is broken forms the foundation of the subsequent doctor–patient relationship. Therefore time invested in this consultation is not wasted.

From their study Kirk and colleagues have distilled six attributes which they found to be important in communicating information:[2]

- honesty
- clarity
- empathy
- time
- pacing of information
- continuity.

The two areas of greatest concern to patients were discussions centred on the issues of *prognosis* and *hope*.

The timing of a discussion about prognosis is important to patients. Some patients have ambivalent views. They may want to be informed of the facts, but at the same time they shrink from knowing the truth. When discussing the prognosis with patients, timing is of paramount importance. Patients often remember the doctor's exact words. This puts an onus on doctors to choose their words carefully. There is often uncertainty when giving a prognosis. The patient may feel more secure if she is given information relevant to her understanding and stage of illness.

Patients want to remain hopeful throughout their illness. Although hope of a miracle cure is remote, assurance of continued support can give confidence into the terminal stages.

Communicating with families

The communication needs of patients and their families change subtly as the illness progresses.[2] During the later stages of the illness, relatives frequently avoid honest communication with the patient and often speak to healthcare providers alone. They often assume that the patient is less aware of his or her situation, an assumption that the study by Kirk and colleagues proved to be false. Patients and their families generally do not talk openly, and tend to shield each other from potentially distressing news. Patients are more concerned with daily living and their symptoms, whereas relatives concentrate on the prognosis and details of care.[2]

A partnership with patients

A partnership is a relationship in which the members work together towards shared goals. A relationship between partners is based on mutual respect, and partners share decision making and responsibility. The key to successful doctor–patient partnerships is to acknowledge that patients also have an area of expertise, namely the patient's own experience of the illness and its effects on psychosocial aspects of their life.[3] There should be provision for patients to share these insights with healthcare professionals, who will then be in a better position to deliver care that is tailored to meet the needs of the individual patient.

The need for information

Research evidence confirms that the vast majority of patients with cancer want to know their diagnosis.[4] In a study of 525 cancer patients, four out of five patients wanted as much information as possible and one in five were not satisfied with the information that they were given. Patients with breast cancer received more information from a wider variety of sources than other cancer patients. Despite this imbalance, the breast cancer patients were no more satisfied than patients with other cancers.[5] Patients wanted more information on the effects of treatment, and on prognosis and recovery. In another study, although patients wanted basic information on diagnosis and treatment, not all of them wanted further information at all stages of their illness.[6] Healthcare professionals frequently underestimate the patient's wish for and ability to cope with information.[7]

Making decisions

Fallowfield has identified two fundamental issues which need to be determined when discussing treatment choices with patients:[8]

1 their own preferences with regard to the amount and type of information that is required
2 their actual rather than perceived desire to participate in decision making.

The desire for information and the wish to take responsibility for decision making are different issues. Some patients may seek information but still prefer the doctor to assume the decision-making role.[9] The challenge facing the doctor is to determine which patients want to be offered choice and which of them would prefer a more passive role. The requirements for informed consent mean that the doctor must use his communication skills to assess what the patient wishes to know and to what extent they wish to take responsibility for decisions that affect their care.

Choice in itself does not prevent psychological morbidity.[10] A study conducted in general practice found that patients felt more secure when seeing a doctor who was known to them and when provided with a longer consultation time.[11] These findings have implications for the provision of personal continuity of care. Patients want to feel empowered to manage their problems.

Quality of life

Quality-of-life measures can reflect the patient's perception of their disease and their preferences for treatment. Many existing quality-of-life measures are standardised and so fail to account for the individual. These measures are therefore applicable to general health status rather than to quality of life.[12] However, it is possible to measure quality of life in a patient-centred way using individualised measures.

Quality of life is determined by the following:[12]

- the extent to which one's expectations are matched by one's experience[13]
- one's perceptions of one's life
- appraisal of one's current state compared with some ideal
- the things that one regards as important.

Quality of life is a dynamic concept that relates to an individual. New measures need to be sophisticated enough to take account of the individual's expectations if they are to help doctors to understand patients' aspirations.

Cultural issues

The cultural beliefs of UK migrants may be very different from those of their doctors. Cultural issues can create communication barriers that can lead to feelings of discrimination and lack of empathy.[14] Those who have grown up in a different culture will have varying traditions, beliefs and values which will affect their response to illness. Coping with cancer in a strange environment that is linguistically and culturally alien may add to the patient's suffering and feeling of isolation. Ethnic minority groups make less use of specialist palliative care resources. Training in communication across cultures is essential if health-care professionals are to engage with ethnic minority patients in a sensitive and professional way.

Patient choice

Patient choice has become a priority on the political agenda. With regard to palliative care this choice means that some patients have the option of remaining at home if local palliative care services and family support are available. Only a small minority have the choice of hospice care. At present patients have a limited choice of professionals who can be involved in their care. Provision of specialist palliative care services is patchy across the UK. Although patients have choices about their management at the end of life, they have no choice as to when that life should end.

Ethics and law

Facilitating choice enhances patient autonomy. However, issues of justice are relevant.

Patients have a legal right to choice:

'An adult patient who suffers from no mental incapacity has an absolute right to choose whether to consent to medical treatment, to refuse it or to choose one rather than another of the treatments being offered.'[15]

They also can refuse any proposed treatment:

'... a person is completely at liberty to decline to undergo treatment ... even if the result of his doing so will be that he will die.'[16]

Doctors have a duty of care not to be negligent and to treat the patient according to his or her best interests. These best interests are not limited to best clinical interests, but include emotional and all other welfare issues.

In *Burke v GMC* the judge ruled that 'the decision as to what is in fact in the patient's best interests is not for the doctor: it is for the patient if competent or, if the patient is incompetent and the matter comes to court, for the judge'.[17]

What is controversial in the Burke case is the idea that a patient may also choose to *require* treatment to be provided even if the doctors have advised against it:

> 'If the patient is competent (or, although incompetent, has made an advance directive ...), his decision to require the provision of artificial nutrition and hydration which he believes is necessary to protect him from what he sees as acute mental and physical suffering is ... in principle determinative.'[17]

Although this ruling was made in relation to a case of artificial nutrition and hydration, its scope and whether it could be applied to all medical decisions is unclear.

When doctors cannot agree to the patient's choice

Doctors are also faced with responding to patients who make a choice to which they cannot agree. For example, in Chapter 11 the case history described a patient who said to her doctor 'Help me to die'. If this request is for euthanasia or physician-assisted suicide, the doctor cannot agree to her choice. This is a difficult request, and the following strategies are suggested for approaching this problem.

Communication strategies

If there is to be effective communication, the patient needs to be able to trust that the doctor has her best interests at heart. The doctor should be willing to follow the patient's concerns and to set aside his own medical agenda.

The patient should be allowed to set the pace of the consultation, and privacy and adequate time must be provided. Effective communication skills should be used, and the doctor should not react immediately, but should pause and acknowledge the request. Protesting that euthanasia is not something that a doctor can carry out blocks any further exploration of the patient's concerns.

The doctor needs to clarify the request without making assumptions. He needs to determine what the patient is really asking for, since a number of possibilities exist. It could be that she is requesting euthanasia, but it is more likely to be a cry for help. Once the doctor begins to explore the background to the request, psychosocial and spiritual dimensions to the problem often emerge. The doctor can show empathy and begin to engage with the patient's suffering. There is no need to suggest any quick solutions. The patient may have misperceptions – for example '*The pain will be terrible*' or '*I am going to be a burden*' – and these should be gently challenged.

Only after he has addressed these concerns should the doctor set boundaries, making it clear that healthcare professionals cannot be involved in euthanasia:

> 'Euthanasia is illegal and I cannot deliberately end your life, but let us look at some of the practical things we can do to help you.'

The euthanasia request is an opportunity to examine what can be done to maximise the patient's dignity and to minimise their suffering.

Although some choices are instinctive, many are based on the patient's assessment of their needs. If doctors cannot agree to that choice, they need to explore those underlying needs and plan the best available means of meeting them so far as is possible within the constraints of the situation.

Promoting choice

Healthcare professionals face the challenge of promoting choice. Eliciting patient preferences, explaining risks and acknowledging uncertainty require good communication skills by all members of the multi-disciplinary team.

This is difficult because patients' preferences change, and their wish to be involved in decision making and the extent of that involvement are hard to assess. There are time constraints because treatment choices are often complex and the patient may not be prepared to assimilate the information during an outpatient clinic appointment. Some patients may opt to forgo their right to choose, and instead ask the doctor to make the treatment decision for them. Limited resources mean that not all patients have an unlimited choice as to where they should be treated and by which provider. Despite these difficulties, doctors need to incorporate discussions about patients' preferences into routine practice.

Key points

- Doctors require the necessary time, communication skills and knowledge of their patients to determine on which occasions and at what level their patients wish to be involved in decision making.
- Ethnic minority groups make less use of specialist palliative care resources than the rest of the population.

- Provision of specialist palliative care services in the UK is patchy.
- A doctor's duty is not to be negligent, and to treat the patient according to his or her best interests.
- Doctors need to incorporate discussions about patients' preferences into routine practice.

References

1 Evans RG (2003) Patient-centred medicine: reason, emotion, and human spirit? Some philosophical reflections on being with patients. *Med Humanities*. **29**: 8–14.
2 Kirk P, Kirk I and Kristjanson LJ (2004) What do patients receiving palliative care for cancer and their families want to be told? A Canadian and Australian qualitative study. *BMJ*. **328**: 1343–7.
3 Coulter A (2002) Patients' views of the good doctor. *BMJ*. **325**: 668–9.
4 Meredith C, Symonds P, Webster L *et al.* (1996) Information needs of cancer patients in west Scotland: cross-sectional survey of patients' views. *BMJ*. **313**: 724–6.
5 Jones R, Pearson J, McGregor S *et al.* (1999) Cross-sectional survey of patients' satisfaction with information about cancer. *BMJ*. **319**: 1247–8.
6 Leydon GM, Boulton M, Moynihan C *et al.* (2000) Cancer patients' information needs and information-seeking behaviour: in-depth interview study. *BMJ*. **320**: 909–13.
7 Jenkins V, Fallowfield L and Saul J (2001) Information needs of patients with cancer: results from a large study in UK cancer centres. *Br J Cancer*. **84**: 48–51.
8 Fallowfield L (2001) Participation of patients in decisions about treatment for cancer. *BMJ*. **323**: 1144.
9 Sutherland HJ, Llewellyn-Thomas HA, Lockwood GA *et al.* (1989) Cancer patients: their desire for information and participation in treatment decisions. *J R Soc Med*. **82**: 260–63.
10 Fallowfield L, Hall A, Maguire P *et al.* (1994) Psychological effects of being offered choice of surgery for breast cancer. *BMJ*. **309**: 448.
11 Howie JGR, Heaney D, Maxwell M *et al.* (1999) Quality of general practice consultations: cross-sectional survey. *BMJ*. **319**: 738–43.
12 Carr AJ and Higginson I (2001) Are quality-of-life measures patient centred? *BMJ*. **322**: 1357–60.
13 Calman KC (1984) Quality of life in cancer patients: a hypothesis. *J Med Ethics*. **10**: 124–7.
14 Eshiett MU-A and Parry EHO (2003) Migrants and health: a cultural dilemma. *Clin Med*. **3**: 229–31.
15 *Re T* [1992] 4 All ER 649 at 652.
16 *Airedale NHS Trust v Bland* [1993] 1 All ER 821.
17 *R (Burke v GMC)* [2004].

13 Communication in multi-disciplinary teams

> The amity that wisdom knits not,
> folly may easily untie.
> *Troilus and Cressida*, III, iii.

Introduction

Patients with advanced life-threatening diseases that are no longer curable have a variety of needs. It is not possible for these needs to be met by a single individual, and multi-disciplinary teamwork is acknowledged to be the most effective model for delivering a high standard of palliative care. The number of professionals involved in a patient's care and the importance of their ability to work collaboratively increases with the complexity of the patient's need.[1] The quality of care depends as much on the sharing of information between professionals as it does on the individual skills of any single member of the multi-disciplinary team.

Case history 1[2]

Ann, a 45-year-old woman, was admitted to hospital with advanced ovarian cancer and multiple liver metastases. The surgeon referred her to the oncologist, who felt that she would not benefit from further chemotherapy. He gave advice on suitable pain control, and as the patient seemed worried, he advised a sedative in addition to her analgesics. Ann was discharged from hospital and referred back to her GP. Unfortunately, her pain was poorly controlled and she died at home three weeks later in some distress.

Case history 2

In the same clinical case, the sequence of referral was similar, except that the surgeons requested a joint assessment by the oncologists and specialist palliative care nurse. During this joint assessment, exploration of Ann's concerns revealed that she was worried she might experience terrible pain. She did not think that her husband would cope on his own, and she felt guilty that she had let him down. The specialist nurse took time to listen to Ann and to address each of these concerns. She then described what resources could be available at home to Ann and her husband. Ann was relieved to hear that her symptom control would be regularly monitored by her GP and district nurse. She was also happy to learn that a specialist palliative care nurse could be involved with the primary care team to support her and her husband.

Ann felt more confident about her discharge home. She was able to talk with her husband about her fears, with the help of a community specialist palliative care nurse. She died at home peacefully three weeks after being discharged from hospital. Six weeks later her husband decided to accept the bereavement support offered by the specialist palliative care nurse.

These two case histories illustrate the variation in quality of life that a patient with advanced cancer may experience as a result of differing communication patterns among healthcare professionals.[2] In both situations the patient died three weeks after discharge from hospital. In the first example, although Ann's physical symptoms were well controlled, neglect of the psychosocial issues meant that she missed an opportunity to resolve unfinished emotional business, and her husband had no bereavement support. In comparison, the second example shows that although Ann had the same short survival, she used this time to come to terms with her fears, and was reassured that her husband would be supported after her death.

Communication between healthcare professionals can be examined at various points during the patient's illness.

Referral

An audit of palliative care at home showed that services were frequently involved too late and that provision of information was often lacking.[3] There was scope for improving teamwork by clarifying roles and sharing information. Delayed referral may result in patients receiving inadequate palliative care. Such delays can result from genuine uncertainties among both patients and healthcare professionals with regard to the role of the palliative care team. Healthcare professionals may also have a sense of vulnerability, or even a desire to protect professional boundaries.

Some doctors believe that specialist palliative care is confined to the terminal phase of the illness, when the patient is obviously dying. However, specialist palliative care teams have emphasised that appropriate referral should be made at an earlier stage in the disease. The decision to refer should be made on the basis of whether the quality of life of patients with advanced disease could be improved and whether they have complex physical or psychosocial needs. Patients and their families need to be fully aware of and in agreement with referral to the specialist palliative care team. This means that the referring doctor or nurse must have a clear understanding of the role of the palliative care team. The professional needs to be comfortable about discussing issues that the patient may raise at the time of this referral. The patient may ask 'Am I going to die?' or perhaps even more difficult questions such as 'Am I going to get better?'.

It is essential that the specialist team liaises with the medical team that is managing the patient, and that the primary team also has full knowledge of and agreement to their involvement. Specialist palliative care is perhaps unusual in that teams accept referrals from a range of fellow healthcare professionals, including doctors or nurses, social workers and professions allied to medicine, as well as self-referral from patients. Many hospital specialist palliative care teams do not take over the complete management of the patient, but share in it as a specialist resource. The specialist team advises and works alongside the primary medical and nursing teams that retain clinical responsibility for the patient. Respect for these professional issues builds trust between teams and allows more flexible inter-professional working.

Palliative care teams have developed referral and eligibility criteria to clarify the process of referral.[4] It is preferable for a letter or an entry in the medical notes requesting a specialist palliative care assessment to confirm verbal referrals. The reason for referral and the degree of urgency should also be specified. The specialist palliative care team should indicate their hours of availability and standard of response.

Multi-disciplinary assessment

An effective multi-disciplinary team relies on good communication between the different professionals involved in care.

Referrals to specialist palliative care teams will be discussed in a multi-disciplinary team meeting and the team will decide which of its members should work together with the patient. The results of the specialist palliative care team assessment are then shared with the primary referring team. This referring team needs to be kept informed of the patient's progress, medication and level of awareness, and about the assessed needs of the family and carers.

Continuing care

Doctors sometimes blame their colleagues for failing to keep them informed about changes occurring in the patient's illness. Information should be passed on with regard to the patient's understanding of the illness and the apparent needs of carers. Responsibility for team success is shared, with balanced participation by team members. In this way conflict can be acknowledged and processed. In a successful team, individual members' roles are defined yet the team works together with shared goals and objectives. Sometimes the effectiveness of the team may be threatened by too much diversity and a lack of communication and coordination.[5] All team members have valuable information to contribute, and the challenge is to achieve information exchange.

Confidentiality

Healthcare professionals have a duty not to divulge information about a patient to a third party without the explicit consent of the patient. A requirement for confidentiality is essential for building a trusting relationship with the patient. However, if multi-disciplinary teamwork is to be effective, information about the patient needs to be shared among members of the team. It is necessary to explain this to the patient and to seek their consent for information to be given to the team. The information can then be shared with other team members on a 'need-to-know' basis. If the patient objects to such disclosures, their right to confidentiality should be respected.[6]

Discharge planning

General practitioners and district nurses are the key professionals responsible for medical and nursing care at home, and they should be the first professionals to be consulted when planning a discharge from hospital. Ideally, when the patient is being discharged the primary care team should be informed about the diagnosis, prognosis, aims of care, treatments, and details of what has been said to the patient and their family. Consensus is necessary between the hospital staff and primary care team on the appropriateness of the discharge and which members of the wider team (e.g. occupational therapists, physiotherapists and social workers) should be involved in care. The social worker coordinates the care at home, involving home care assistance, the primary care team, specialist palliative care services and non-professional voluntary support. Discharge information must be sent promptly to the GP. GPs do not want to give conflicting messages or be ignorant of the facts when facing patients and their relatives at this critical time.

Anecdotal evidence exists of inter-professional rivalries and poor communication between healthcare professionals.[7] Failure of teamwork may be due to a lack of common objectives, ignorance of respective roles and professional insecurity.

End-of-life and terminal care

Ethical dilemmas do not have easy answers, and reaching a moral consensus in the team is often difficult. It is a necessary part of good clinical practice to ensure that everyone concerned is given a chance to express their own views. Nurses work closely with patients, and doctors need to listen to their views before making decisions.

Bereavement support

In bereavement care the roles of the doctor, nurse, social worker and health visitor are complementary. Voluntary organisations, clergy and palliative care teams may also be sources of support to the bereaved. Effective communication between the professionals is as important at this stage as it is during the earlier phases of the patient's illness. There must be an efficient means of notifying the GP and the primary care team of the patient's death. This avoids the embarrassing error of a member of the team visiting the patient's home in ignorance of the death, and it ensures that the GP or community nurse can offer bereavement support.

Barriers to effective inter-professional communication

In palliative care, effective communication between healthcare professionals may be impaired for a number of reasons.

- Palliative care is provided in diverse settings – home, community hospital, nursing home, hospice and hospital.
- Specialist palliative care teams often work at the interface between curative and palliative care.
- Specialist palliative care teams have to liaise between different teams of healthcare professionals, and voluntary and statutory agencies.
- Respect for confidentiality may hamper frank discussion between team members.

Communication issues

Healthcare systems may become inefficient due to poor communication infrastructures in practice. An Australian survey of hospital admissions found that a lack of communication was the commonest cause of preventable disability or death.[8]

Communication mechanisms may be either synchronous, when two individuals participate in a conversation at the same time (which tends to be interruptive), or asynchronous, when the exchange does not require both individuals to be active participants at the same time, so the receiver can choose the moment to reply.

Shared communication can result in an interruptive workplace and contribute to inefficiency. The psychological costs associated with interruption can cause diversion of attention, forgetfulness and errors. Such interruptions may result in rescheduling of work plans. Doctors may not consider the effect that a telephone call or pager has on the other party, perhaps valuing the completion of their own tasks over that of their colleagues. Regular meetings are necessary between the doctor and nurse to allow the handing over of details of the patient's progress, drug changes and any communications between the professional and the patient or family. Effective communication between nurses and doctors is enhanced by the formation of good interpersonal relationships, in which nurses feel able to communicate their feelings about their patients without fear of ridicule by medical colleagues.

Communication and conflict

Conflict should be acknowledged using a problem-solving approach. Unsatisfactory communication lies at the heart of many of the stresses experienced by professionals working in palliative care. Complaints from patients may be generated by a criticism of a general practitioner by hospital staff. Concerns about patient care should be discussed with the colleague in private in the first instance, not in front of the patient.

Palliative care must embrace uncertainty in cases where decisions are made with inadequate information and where there may be conflicting advice from colleagues. Such uncertainty needs to be acknowledged among doctors and their colleagues. Ethical dilemmas can be a source of stress, which can be diffused by calling a family meeting or case conference to reach a team consensus. Clinical supervision, mentoring and peer appraisal are all methods of supporting and encouraging colleagues.

Improving communication

Appropriate referral to a specialist team should be made whenever a healthcare professional reaches the limits of their own skills. The introduction of clinical governance has placed more emphasis on ensuring that patients receive appropriate care.

Team members need instruction in the appropriate use of communication facilities. Voicemail, email and mobile phone communication can improve support. Healthcare professionals should consider the consequences of communication action with regard to their colleagues, and reflect on the use of resources. Joint consultations may be facilitated by teleconferencing through sound and video links without having to leave the workplace.

Education

General Medical Council guidance on maintaining good medical practice states that one of the key tests of a good team is that the members can be 'open and honest about professional performance'. This requires a willingness to engage directly across boundaries that have long been impermeable.[9] An important objective of inter-professional education is the fostering of mutual respect. Common training programmes in communication skills also challenge working practices. Although updates of clinical knowledge for individual doctors remain important, further learning is needed on multi-disciplinary working.

GPs who in the past tended to work independently need to embrace multi-professional teamworking, readily enlisting the skills and knowledge of a specialist palliative care team.

Doctors and nurses have essentially different professional training, and there is therefore a possibility that their views may become entrenched, thereby hampering effective teamwork. If doctors and nurses were to receive some aspects of their education together, this might help to remove barriers. GPs and hospital consultants have a high level of mutual respect and cooperation, and most branches of the profession try hard to avoid potential conflict.

Improved records

Patient-held records are useful when moving from one setting to another. They improve continuity, awareness and understanding of the different roles of participating healthcare professionals. Their use may also encourage partnership in care and facilitate open exchanges between patients and healthcare professionals. Electronic communications may unite practices and hospital trusts, thereby reducing paperwork and speeding up access to results, hospital referrals and discharge letters by the use of email.

Conclusions

Collaborative practice involves good communication within a team. Individuals and groups depend on each other for information and help, and their interdependence may result in either a competitive or a collaborative relationship. Inter-professional education results in improved understanding of professional roles in collaborative working. Patients and their families will benefit if physicians are aware of their own skills and limitations and are ready to employ the skills of others. Continuity of care builds trust, and this facilitates the introduction of other healthcare professionals into a patient's care. The physician who is involved with the patient over time is in the best position to initiate a team approach. The initial implementation of a team approach often hinges on the doctor's recognition of the need for an inter-disciplinary approach to care. A team of reliable professionals provides patients with a sense of security, consistency and comfort. In an effective and efficient inter-disciplinary team, each member will have an understanding of the roles of the other members.

Many of the stresses reported by healthcare professionals when caring for the dying are not a direct result of working with the patient or their family but a consequence of difficulties with colleagues and institutional hierarchies.

Key points

- Inter-disciplinary teamwork is acknowledged to be the most effective model for delivery of a high standard of palliative care.
- The decision to refer to specialist palliative care services should be based on whether the quality of life of patients with advanced disease could be improved.
- The quality of inter-disciplinary teamwork is dependent on a complex process of sharing clinical, emotional and social assessments between the different professionals, the carers and the patients.
- Appropriate referral to a specialist team should be made whenever a healthcare professional reaches the limits of their own skills.
- One of the key tests of a good team is that its members can be open and honest about professional performance.

References

1 Headrick LA, Wilcock PM and Batalden PB (1998) Interprofessional working and continuing medical education. *BMJ*. **316**: 711–14.
2 Coyle N (1997) Interdisciplinary collaboration in hospital palliative care: chimera or goal? *Palliat Med*. **11**: 265–6.
3 Miller DG, Carroll D, Grimshaw J *et al.* (1998) Palliative care at home: an audit of cancer deaths in the Grampian region. *Br J Gen Pract*. **48**: 1299–302.
4 Bennett M, Adam J, Alison D *et al.* (2000) Leeds eligibility criteria for specialist palliative care services. *Palliat Med*. **14**: 157–8.
5 Mystakidou K (2001) Interdisciplinary working: a Greek perspective. *Palliat Med*. **15**: 67–8.
6 Doyle D and Jeffrey D (2000) *Palliative Care in the Home*. Oxford University Press, Oxford.
7 Black OJ (1996) Supportive and shared care. In: BO Hancock (ed.) *Cancer Care in the Community* (9e). Radcliffe Medical Press, Oxford.
8 Coiera E and Tombs V (1998) Communication behaviour in a hospital setting: an observational study. *BMJ*. **316**: 673–6.
9 General Medical Council (2001) *Good Medical Practice*. General Medical Council, London.

14 Education, ethics and communication skills

Happy are they that hear their detractions and can
Put them to mending.

Much Ado About Nothing, II, iii.

Introduction

A team approach is the optimal model of delivery of palliative care, yet health-care professionals' education still tends to occur within single disciplines. It would be more appropriate to adopt a multi-disciplinary approach to the teaching of and training in ethics and communication skills, to reflect clinical practice.[1]

Healthcare professionals may feel inhibited about teaching ethics and communication skills for a number of reasons.[2] Some clinicians have little teaching experience and lack confidence in their ability to teach, especially a complex topic such as ethics. Time may also be a constraint – in a busy clinical schedule there is little protected time for education.

Ethics and communication are sensitive areas, and there is rarely one right answer. Teaching and learning should take place in an environment in which everyone's view is respected and where a positive approach is emphasised – a culture of 'positive critique'. Praise and constructive criticism are much more effective teaching tools than humiliation.

In such a learning situation people feel confident to disclose areas of difficulty. This type of environment facilitates the development of healthcare professionals who are both competent and compassionate, and who are inspired to continue to develop their own education. Education should be liberating, yet sometimes disturbing, affecting both practice and experience.

The teaching approach

When planning any educational programme the learners' needs should be established. Knowles has identified seven principles of adult learning that need to be addressed by teachers:[3]

1 Establish a physical and psychological climate or ethos of learning.
2 Involve learners in mutual planning and curriculum directions.
3 Involve learners in diagnosing their own needs.
4 Involve learners in formulating their own learning objectives.
5 Involve learners in identifying resources and devising strategies using those resources to accomplish their objectives.
6 Help learners to carry out their learning plans.
7 Involve learners in evaluating their learning, principally through qualitative evaluation methods.

These principles facilitate a shift of responsibility for change to the learner.

A 'good' teacher?

The qualities of a 'good' teacher relate closely to those of a 'good' doctor and a 'good' person. Common virtues identified in good teachers include the following:

- enthusiasm
- friendliness
- an interest in students and learners
- competence
- knowledge
- confidence
- charisma
- willingness to prepare well
- patience
- ability to listen.

Perhaps the most important ability is to make the learner feel valued by respecting his or her views. Teachers are facilitators rather than transmitters of facts. Teaching and learning are complementary – the good teacher is always willing to learn from the student.

The learning environment

The aim of the teaching is to produce practitioners who are both scientifically competent and sensitive to the (often unspoken) needs of patients and their families. Teachers must provide a role model, show that they are flexible and be committed to a team approach. Teamworking is adaptable and non-hierarchical, and leadership is necessary to give direction but can change according to the teaching situation. Teachers and learners set their objectives together. Teaching is firmly rooted in clinical practice so that learners can grasp the relevance of the material to their work. Teaching in this way is not a passive transmission of knowledge, but rather it is an active problem-solving process. By using interactive methods and engaging learners in their own education, those learners are motivated to understand and reflect on the relevance of ethics and communication skills. Interactive teaching involves the learners in critically evaluating their own beliefs and values. In this way they can enhance their professional judgements in clinical situations which can be filled with uncertainty. To function effectively in this environment, healthcare professionals need to have the confidence to share difficulties with colleagues, making professional decisions despite the complexity of the situation and the uncertainty of the outcome.

Planning

The success of a clinical intervention will often depend on the time and care taken during the initial assessment. The success of a teaching session also depends on the time and care taken in planning. There should be negotiation with learners to set aims for the programme, while at the same time retaining a willingness to adapt the plan during the course of the teaching session.

Choice of teaching technique

Teachers select a variety of teaching techniques in advance which will encourage participation by the whole group – for example, an opening 'icebreaker' which is an activity involving everyone in the group. If the session is on communication skills, the teacher needs to decide whether a teaching video or role play would be more appropriate. Time needs to be allocated for discussion and reflection, and fewer subjects should be studied rather than rushing through a busy agenda at the risk of confusing students. Facilitators should be aware that participants may become distressed, and should be ready to change the agenda if this happens.

Teaching formats

Teaching formats vary. Some of the most commonly used formats for ethics and communication skills include small group teaching, tutorials, clinical 'bedside', supervision and debate. In order to develop a learner's ethical sensitivity and communication skills, the teaching format must encourage reflection on their own clinical experience.

Teaching techniques

It is beyond the scope of this chapter to cover all teaching techniques, but a few crucial points may be emphasised which have particular relevance for teaching ethics and communication skills.

Ground rules

Ground rules are an agreed set of conditions that the group negotiates and abides by. Their purpose is to allow people to feel confident, secure and relaxed in an optimal learning environment. People neither take in nor retain new information if they are anxious or apprehensive. Ground rules enable a safe trusting environment to be created in which learners can reflect on their own beliefs, values and attitudes without feeling threatened. Confidentiality and respect for the opinions of others are essential. Participants also feel more comfortable if they have explicit permission to call 'time out'. Positive critique means that in any situation participants must identify things that are going well before any suggestions are made as to how a situation could be improved. It is important to set such ground rules in any small group or interactive session in which people are exploring sensitive issues or where there is a potential for self-disclosure.

Icebreakers

One of the greatest barriers to effective communication is the natural reticence of participants about contributing, particularly at the outset of a teaching event. An icebreaker is an activity that aims to promote participation by all members of the group. Group members are allowed a degree of self-disclosure in order to get to know each other better.

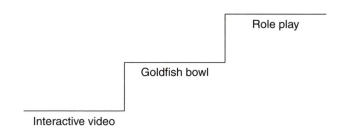

Figure 14.1 Communication Skills Ladder

The Communication Skills Ladder

Communication skills can be taught using a variety of techniques that enable learners to practise these skills in situations that are as close to those encountered in real life as possible. Many participants feel inhibited about practising their communication skills. One way of overcoming this difficulty is to use the Communication Skills Ladder (*see* Figure 14.1).

The first step in the ladder involves interactive and experiential work that is non-threatening. At the next step the degree of personal participation increases, as does the potential for the learner to feel threatened. If communication skills are to improve, it is necessary for the participants to feel confident enough to practise their skills and to receive constructive feedback from colleagues.

Interactive video

Interactive videos that are used as a first step in practising communication skills involve actors and actresses playing the roles of clinicians and patients. The learners may participate in this activity. When the facilitator has stopped the tape he prompts the group to offer positive critique on the skills displayed by the clinician. The tape is then restarted in order to follow the story. Such videos are useful in a number of situations – for example, with a group of individuals who do not know each other, or with students who do not have their own reservoir of experiences upon which to draw.

Goldfish bowl

The goldfish bowl technique involves the learners observing the teaching team performing a role play. A facilitator stops the role play and the learners are then asked to contribute suggestions concerning what language the role players might use to deal with a communication problem. They then watch as their suggestions are enacted in the role play. This allows participants to contribute their own ideas on different approaches without feeling threatened by actually having to take part in a role play themselves.

Role play

In role play, participants or facilitators take on the roles of patients, families and healthcare professionals and enact a situation. This is a useful way of practising communication skills in a safe environment without upsetting patients. Role play is used in small group settings with participants who are comfortable practising their communication skills. It can also be used with larger groups, which can be divided into pairs or trios. Some people may have already practised other techniques in the Communication Skills Ladder, but want an opportunity to practise their skills among themselves.

Evaluation

Evaluation measures the effectiveness of the educational process, one component of which is the performance of the teacher. It is quite distinct from assessment, which measures the attainments and achievements of learners in terms of their knowledge, skills and attitudes.

Evaluation of an education programme is undertaken by both teachers and students. When reflecting on the programme, teachers and students evaluate how effectively each prepared for the session, how needs were met and whether sufficient time was allowed.

Arts and humanities

The aim of teaching the humanities within medical education is to provide an opportunity to see the world from another person's point of view. It enables doctors to embrace uncertainty and to improve their communication skills in clinical practice.[4,5]

The arts may stimulate insight into both shared experiences and individual differences. They can also enrich the language and thoughts of healthcare professionals. If doctors and nurses are to be both competent and compassionate, the arts as well as the sciences should be included in medical training.

Art as language

The visual arts can be used as a medium to improve communication skills, moving away from the usual channels of the written word to explore the nature of human experience. Looking outside conventional communication structures generates a more spontaneous response, bringing the doctor closer to sharing the patient's perspective. The group is involved in looking at and responding spontaneously to various pictures. Such an activity in a teaching environment is a new experience for many healthcare professionals.

Knowledge of the patient's diagnosis or social circumstances cannot in itself inform us of their outlook, understanding or beliefs. There is a wide range of individual responses to experience, yet little emphasis is placed on this in traditional healthcare training.

Medical practitioners who appreciate and learn from the arts gain a greater understanding of the human condition. By looking at pieces of artwork and examining the range of reactions that exist among colleagues, participants become more aware of the individuality of responses. The clinical benefits of this process should include improved communication skills and more effective problem solving.

Storytelling and narrative medicine

Storytelling and narrative medicine have been used to develop a patient-centred approach to ethics and communication. This can take many forms (e.g. creative writing, storytelling in small groups, reflective portfolios and group role plays), all of which bring another perspective to the medical world. Stories can develop empathy and understanding of the patient's perspective. Although knowledge acquired from scientific evidence is given the highest value in medicine, much can also be learned from stories and anecdotes, provided that 'we are prepared to listen'.[6] To learn through storytelling is to recognise the human need to create meaning from experience.[7]

Conclusion

The teaching of ethics and communication skills aims to inspire healthcare professionals to think, reflect and improve their professional judgement. Education is a process of facilitation whereby the teacher recognises the potential within the learner and inspires the desire to learn. The learner becomes responsible for his or her own education, and in learning seeks to understand. It is this understanding which is of ultimate value in education.

If effective learning is to take place, an environment is needed in which experienced professionals can express their doubts and feelings of vulnerability without feeling inadequate. Experience is at the heart of adult learning, and learners bring their own skills and perspectives which enrich the learning environment.[8]

The good teacher ascertains the learner's needs and negotiates clear learning objectives. This emphasis on the relevance of teaching material is reflected in modern 'problem-orientated' curricula in medical schools.

Learners flourish in an environment facilitated by enthusiastic teachers with a philosophy of positive critique. They become reflective practitioners who are willing to examine their knowledge, attitudes and experience.

Working with uncertainty requires professionals to listen to others and adopt a flexible approach, ready to make professional judgements when there is no right answer. 'Practical wisdom' is this combination of empathy and clinical competence.

References

1 Keogh K, Jeffrey D and Flanagan S (1999) The Palliative Care Education Group for Gloucestershire (PEGG): an integrated model of multidisciplinary education in palliative care. *Eur J Cancer Care.* **8**: 44–7.
2 Jeffrey D (ed.) (2002) *Teaching Palliative Care: a practical guide.* Radcliffe Medical Press, Oxford.
3 Knowles MS (1984) *Andragogy in Action: applying modern principles of adult learning.* Jossey-Bass, San Francisco, CA.
4 Jeffrey D, Jeffrey P, Jones D and Owen R (2001) An innovative, practical course in the medical humanities. *Eur J Palliat Care.* **8**: 5.
5 General Medical Council (1993) *Tomorrow's Doctors.* General Medical Council, London.
6 Macnaughton J (1995) Anecdotes and empiricism. *Br J Gen Pract.* **Nov**: 571.
7 Alterio M (2002) *Reflective learning through storytelling.* Paper presented at Institute for Learning and Teaching in Higher Education Annual Conference, Edinburgh, 2002.
8 Newman P and Peile E (2002) Valuing learners' experience and supporting further growth: educational models to help experienced adult learners in medicine. *BMJ.* **325**: 200–2.

15 The 'good' doctor: a virtue-based approach to ethics

He lives in fame that died in virtue's cause.
Titus Andronicus, I, i.

Virtue ethics

The central question in ethics is 'How should I live?' Ethics is concerned with concepts of good conduct – with the nature and justification of principles of behaviour. There have been numerous attempts to define the virtues that make up the 'good' doctor. By exploring these virtues, it is hoped that common themes that define this elusive concept may emerge. However, it may prove difficult to differentiate between a 'good' doctor and a 'good' human being.

Virtue ethics describes an approach to ethics that emphasises the virtues rather than duties or rules (deontology) or consequences of actions (utilitarianism). Virtue ethics dates back to Plato and Aristotle and involves a discussion of issues such as motives, moral character, moral wisdom, relationships and emotions.[1]

When considering medical practice, virtue ethics provides a different framework, in which concern is directed towards identifying and nurturing the virtues that characterise a good person, rather than an approach based on ethical principles.

Virtues

Virtues are character traits that lead to consistency of actions. They are more than tendencies to act in a certain way, and once acquired they become a habit.[1] For example, when seeking informed consent, a doctor who has the virtue of honesty tells the truth and ensures that the patient really understands the issues. Such a doctor would defend the importance of trust in the doctor–patient relationship.

Aristotle described the virtues as 'excellences' of character, each involving *phronesis* or practical wisdom. Practical wisdom is the ability to reason correctly about practical matters. A virtue is something that makes a person good, so a virtuous person is someone who is morally good and who also acts well. A virtue is a character trait that can satisfy the human need for *eudaimonia*, which means to flourish or live well.

There has been some dispute about which character traits are virtues. Classical Aristotelian virtues include justice, honesty, charity, courage, practical wisdom, generosity and loyalty. In describing the virtues of a 'good' doctor, different traits might be listed – for example, humility, competence, compassion and tolerance.

How can virtues help us to understand practical ethics?

Virtue ethics poses the question 'What sort of person should I be?'. It is considered to be an 'agent-centred' rather than an 'act-centred' type of ethics. How then does virtue ethics provide guidance on how we should behave? Hursthouse maintains that virtue ethics defines right action as 'what a virtuous person would characteristically do in the circumstances'. Thus virtue ethics can generate rules and principles, since each virtue generates an instruction ('do what is honest') and each vice generates a prohibition ('do not act in a dishonest way').[1]

Many of the end-of-life ethical dilemmas that were discussed in previous chapters have no one 'right' answer, and definite guidance for action cannot be laid down. However, virtue ethics can provide guidance for an ethical *assessment* of the issues, enabling decisions to be made that incorporate emotions into the ethical decision. Virtues are concerned with both actions and feelings.

When virtues conflict

The diverse requirements of virtues can pull in different directions. For example, in a particular case it may be considered compassionate to kill a person who would 'be better off dead', but a sense of justice prevents this from happening. To be honest demands that the truth be told, but in a case where a patient might suffer harm, compassion may cause the healthcare professional to remain silent.

Can virtue ethics help with really difficult moral quandaries?

Virtue ethics takes into account feelings such as regret, guilt or sorrow in the ethical assessment. Patients often complain not about the decision but about the manner in which it was communicated – for example, if the doctor appears arrogant or does not express regret. Virtue ethics makes the doctor concentrate on the manner as well as the content of his or her response.

A doctor may ask 'What is the morally correct decision for me to make here?'. Virtues cannot be ranked in order of priority, as there will always be particular circumstances in a dilemma that generate exceptions to any 'rule'. Moral wisdom is a combination of knowledge, life experience and humanity, and is demonstrated by exercising one's judgement. In difficult situations, virtue ethics requires the doctor to seek moral guidance from a more experienced, wiser colleague.

Irresolvable dilemmas

An irresolvable dilemma is a situation in which the doctor's choice lies between two alternatives and there are no moral reasons for favouring one course of action over the other.[1] Utilitarian theory tries to eliminate the dilemma through a calculation of the greatest happiness for the greatest number. Deontologists reject that calculation and attempt to capture the complexity of real-life dilemmas with a list of rules and principles.

Perhaps it is more honest to admit that there are distressing dilemmas for which there is no single 'right' answer. Proponents of virtue ethics accept the possibility of irresolvable dilemmas because they accept that a fixed decision procedure cannot be found. Faced with the same moral choice, two virtuous people can act differently and still both be assessed as 'acting well'.

Irresolvable dilemmas and virtue ethics

An irresolvable dilemma might be whether to discontinue artificial feeding and hydration in an unconscious patient with terminal cancer. Virtue ethics allows for the possibility that two virtuous relatives faced with the same decision in the same circumstances may act differently – one opts for asking the doctors to continue treatment while the other asks them to discontinue it.

These two individuals are equally virtuous without having exactly the same standards and ideals. One relative says 'I must accept that my mother is mortal', while the other thinks 'I mustn't give up hope'. From a virtue ethics perspective they each 'acted well' – that is, courageously, thoughtfully, honestly and wisely.

In difficult cases there are situations where the doctor may experience feelings of regret, sorrow or guilt. Virtue ethics provides insights into why decisions are difficult, justifies the need to accept advice and explains the existence of irresolvable dilemmas. However, great care should be taken to avoid labelling every difficult dilemma as necessarily 'irresolvable'.

Emotion and motivation

Emotions are an unreliable source of acting well – they need to be regulated by *phronesis* or practical wisdom. Sympathy, compassion and love are emotions that promote the good of others. However, there may be a risk of paternalism on the part of a doctor who assumes that he knows the feelings of the patient. Misconception of a good may make someone act wrongly. For example, misguided compassion may prompt a doctor to lie because he feels that the patient will not wish to know the hurtful truth of his condition. There may even be a vanity in wanting to be the 'special person' who helps the patient.

Emotions are morally significant

Virtues are traits not only to act but also to feel emotions. Such emotions may initiate an action or be the consequence of such an action.

Although Kant considered that emotions are no part of our rationality, the

Stoics felt that the emotions are part of our rational nature and that they influence judgement. The emotion that enables animals to be aware of danger can be transformed in human beings into an emotion connected with the preservation of what is best.[1]

In palliative care a value is placed on 'being there' for other people, where patients talk of their suffering. Doctors experience emotions of sadness or powerlessness, as there may be nothing that they can do to 'make it better'. Any comfort that they are able to provide stems from their emotional reactions, and if the doctor fails to make this appropriate response they have failed to meet the patient's need, and this is a moral failure.[1]

In palliative care, doctors also have needs and emotions of their own – a sense of failure, grief or anger, or a desire to avoid the patient in order to escape these feelings.[2] Doctors should address their emotions using a process of reflection and self-monitoring. For example, the following four steps can help doctors to cope with their feelings.

1 Name the emotion.
2 Accept the normality of the feeling.
3 Reflect on the emotion and its consequences.
4 Consult a wise and trusted colleague.[2]

Such a process may form part of reflective practice or mentoring.

Moral motivation

The virtuous doctor is morally motivated and acts from a settled state of good character with the appropriate intentions, feelings and attitudes.[1] In general, virtue is a complex sensitivity, an ability to recognise the requirements that situations impose on one's behaviour.[3]

The virtues of the 'good doctor': the professionals' view

The General Medical Council (GMC) has listed its requirements of a good doctor (*see* Chapter 4, p. 41).[4] These duties encompass virtues such as altruism, courage, politeness, respect, honesty, competence and fairness. They strive to combine the skills of an applied scientist with the attributes of a wise reflective practitioner.[5] The GMC emphasises the importance of doctors being open to learning from their mistakes. In the UK there have recently been a number of high-profile inquiries into the practice of both individuals and hospital trusts. As a result, the GMC is in the process of reviewing its guidance document *Good Medical Practice*. In some situations it may be the organisation of health-care which is at fault rather than any individual doctor.

However, a distinction should be drawn between the practice of medicine and an organisation such as a hospital trust. The practice of medicine has a history – it involves standards of excellence and obedience to rules as well as the achievement of good. To enter medical practice is to accept the authority of those standards and to subject one's own attitudes, choices and preferences to the standards that currently define the practice. These standards can be criticised, but they are the best that can be devised at present. Medical practice requires a certain kind of relationship between those who participate in it, which encompasses virtues such as justice, courage, care and truthfulness.[6]

Medical professionalism

Professionalism is the basis of medicine's contract with society. It demands that the interests of patients be placed above those of the doctor, as well as the setting and maintaining of standards of competence, integrity, and providing society with expert advice on matters of health.[7] Public trust forms the basis of this contract, as society's need for the healer and its belief in the inherent virtue and morality of professionalism serve as the basis of medicine.[8]

Professionalism is based on three fundamental principles:

1 the primacy of patient welfare
2 patient autonomy
3 social justice.

Doctors tend to focus on personal qualities more than on knowledge and technical skills when describing a good doctor. Some have suggested that in view of the uncertainties of practice it may be sufficient to strive to be 'good enough' practitioners.[5] Virtues such as conscience and self-reflection may not guarantee 'goodness in doctors' – hence the need for systems of appraisal and revalidation.

There is a risk that compliance with guidelines will become a measure of the 'goodness' of practitioners. Once competence and performance have been verified, it is difficult to define the remaining traits that are integral to the concept of a 'good' doctor. In relation to medicine the term 'good' often means that the doctor has passed tests of competency. Such tests may not detect poor doctors.

Good communication skills are an essential part of a 'good' doctor. Moreover, these skills can be developed through teaching and training.[9] Doctors who allow the patient to tell their story without interruption elicit more information and patient satisfaction without extending the total visit time.[10]

Students seek role models who display virtues of enthusiasm, compassion, openness, integrity and good communication with patients. However, such role models may not be able to communicate professional attitudes and behaviours, and poor attitudes displayed by their senior colleagues cause distress and anger in young doctors.[11]

What do patients think?

Despite adverse publicity in recent years, most patients trust doctors.[12] Patients want a good interpersonal relationship and a high standard of technical care from their doctors. In a recent systematic review of the European literature, the following themes emerged: humaneness, competency, time for care and patient involvement in decision making.[13] Many of the public's unfulfilled expectations of doctors are about attitudes. Patients want doctors to acknowledge that:

- good communication is essential
- patients can choose treatment options
- patronising or arrogant behaviour is unacceptable
- poor practice should be confronted in an open manner
- doctors should be accountable
- the profession should punish misconduct.[14]

Conclusions

Doctors and patients do not always agree on priorities. Patients need empathy, support, reassurance, honest information and clinicians who will listen to their concerns.

Time should be devoted in undergraduate curricula to developing appropriate professional behaviour. Innovative teaching techniques such as mentoring, the use of the arts and humanities and group discussions can give students and young doctors the opportunity to develop an ethical sensitivity and effective communication skills. All doctors need to examine their values, attitudes and behaviour from the viewpoint of their patients. Looking through others' eyes is a good starting point for morality.

References

1 Hursthouse R (1999) *On Virtue Ethics*. Oxford University Press, Oxford.
2 Meier DE, Back AL and Morrison S (2001) The inner life of physicians and care of the seriously ill. *JAMA*. **286**: 3007–14.
3 McDowell J (2003) Virtue and reason. In: S Darwall (ed.) *Virtue Ethics*. Blackwell Publishing, Oxford.
4 General Medical Council (2001) *Good Medical Practice*. General Medical Council, London.
5 Hurwitz B and Vass A (2002) What's a good doctor, and how can you make one? *BMJ*. **325**: 667–8.
6 MacIntyre A (2003) The nature of the virtues. In: S Darwall (ed.) *Virtue Ethics*. Blackwell Publishing, Oxford.
7 Medical Professionalism Project (2002) Medical professionalism in the new millennium: a physician's charter. *Clin Med JRCPL*. **2**: 116–18.
8 Cruess RL, Cruess SR and Johnston SE (2000) Professionalism: an ideal to be sustained. *Lancet*. **356**: 156–9.
9 Maguire P and Pitceathley C (2002) Key communication skills and how to acquire them. *BMJ*. **325**: 697–700.
10 Mechanic D (2002) Managing time appropriately in primary care. *BMJ*. **325**: 690.
11 Paice E, Heard S and Moss F (2002) How important are role models in making good doctors? *BMJ*. **325**: 707–10.
12 Coulter A (2002) Patients' views of the good doctor. *BMJ*. **325**: 668–9.
13 Wensing M, Jung HP, Mainz J *et al*. (1998) A systematic review of the literature on patient priorities for general practice care. Part 1. Description of the research domain. *Soc Sci Med*. **47**: 1573–88.
14 Irvine D (1999) The performance of doctors: the new professionalism. *Lancet*. **353**: 1174–7.

Conclusion: learning to listen

Palliative care faces the challenge of integrating with mainstream medicine yet retaining its holistic ethos. It developed as a response to the concept of 'total pain', and psychosocial care ensures that it continues to engage with suffering. A 'good' death can be achieved, but there is a need for political institutions and primary care trusts to acknowledge this as a priority.

Ethics and communication permeate every aspect of palliative care. In seeking to maximise the patient's quality of life such care places value on patient autonomy. Autonomy is not simply individual independence. It demands integrity, responsibility and critical reflection on the part of the individual. In providing care for the relatives as well as the patient, palliative care acknowledges this broad view of autonomy.

Clinical situations at the end of life can create ethical dilemmas. A review of ethical models demonstrates the value of taking an 'ethical pause' before making a decision. Eventually decisions have to be made, and effective communication can ensure that all those involved make the best possible choice. Ethics is a discipline that involves both communication and emotion in its application to clinical care. Models of virtue ethics and responsibility ethics have a special relevance to end-of-life care.

Communication is central to palliative care. Doctors with an awareness of the barriers to good communication can practise more effectively. When informed of a recurrence of their cancer, patients make realistic treatment choices if they are given honest information. A requirement for informed and understood consent protects patients from well-intentioned paternalism. It is legitimate for a patient to ask a doctor what he considers to be the best course of action. To abandon patients who seek guidance for their decisions is not to respect their autonomy. Consent procedures are necessary to moderate the pace of scientific research, and this protection is of particular relevance in palliative care.

Doctors' skills in delivering bad news are improving, but there is a need for further training in areas relating to communication of the risks of treatments. There is much rhetoric supporting communication skills training, but in practice little takes place, due to competing clinical responsibilities and a lack of resources.

Ethical dilemmas encountered at the end of life often relate to the withdrawal or withholding of treatments – for example, chemotherapy, cardiac resuscitation or hydration. Joint working between oncology and palliative care services can lead to collaborative practice in these areas. Lack of competence is being addressed by legislation. In future, proxy decision making and advance directives may help to clarify the doctor's dilemmas.

The legalisation of euthanasia has recently been considered in the House of Lords, and the Select Committee reflected the public division into two camps. There is a need to accept that this is an irresolvable issue and to seek better ways of dealing with unrelieved suffering. A solution would be to resource palliative care so that all patients had access to a good standard of such care. Education could play an important role in helping patients and the public to achieve their choices by advance planning for their deaths. Healthcare professionals need to be comfortable when talking to patients about end-of-life care. Patient choice has become a political mantra, but many of the 'choices' are illusory, as not all patients can obtain palliative care, and very few have access to hospice care.

Healthcare professionals should strive to make care of the patient the focus of their attention. The majority of healthcare professionals work most effectively in multi-disciplinary teams rather than striving to protect professional boundaries.

Ethical behaviour and effective communication require doctors to reflect on their practice and to learn from patients. To see the world through the eyes of the individual patient enables the doctor to deliver effective clinical care.

Index

Page numbers in *italics* refer to figures.